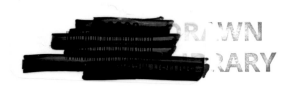
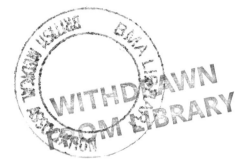
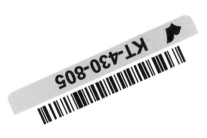

INTRODUCTION TO

ORGAN
TRANSPLANTATION

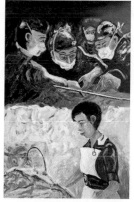

2nd Edition

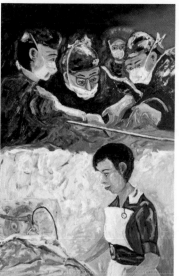

INTRODUCTION TO
ORGAN
TRANSPLANTATION

2nd Edition

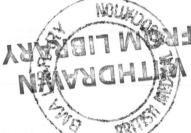

Edited by

Nadey S Hakim

Imperial College Healthcare NHS Trust, London, UK

Foreword by

David Taube

Imperial College Healthcare NHS Trust, London, UK

Imperial College Press

Published by

Imperial College Press
57 Shelton Street
Covent Garden
London WC2H 9HE

Distributed by

World Scientific Publishing Co. Pte. Ltd.
5 Toh Tuck Link, Singapore 596224
USA office: 27 Warren Street, Suite 401-402, Hackensack, NJ 07601
UK office: 57 Shelton Street, Covent Garden, London WC2H 9HE

British Library Cataloguing-in-Publication Data
A catalogue record for this book is available from the British Library.

INTRODUCTION TO ORGAN TRANSPLANTATION
2nd Edition

ISBN-13 978-1-84816-854-1
ISBN-10 1-84816-854-3

Typeset by Stallion Press
Email: enquiries@stallionpress.com

Printed in Singapore by Mainland Press Pte Ltd.

If we excel in anything, it is in our capacity for translating idealism into action.

Charles H Mayo, MD

Dedicated to my children: David, Alexandra, Andrea and Gabi.

Contents

Contributors

Miss Christina D. Bali MD PhD
Transplant Fellow
The West London Renal and Transplant Centre,
Hammersmith Hospital, London

Mr Ruben Canelo MD FICS FRCS FACS FEBS
Consultant HPB and Transplant Surgeon,
Buenos Aires, Argentina

Professor Jacques Colombani MD
Professor of Medicine
Centre d'ettude du Polymorphisme Humain (CEPH), Paris

Mr Dai M. Davies FRCS
Plastic, Reconstructive & Aesthetic Surgeon, Director
Institute of Cosmetic & Reconstructive Surgery,
West London Clinic, London

Dr Miran Epstein MD PhD MA
Reader in Medical Ethics and Law
Barts and The London School of Medicine and Dentistry,
Queen Mary, University of London, London

Professor Nadey S. Hakim MD PhD FRCS FACS FICS
Consultant Surgeon, Surgical Director,
The West London Renal and Transplant Centre,
Hammersmith Hospital, London

Mr Nicos Kessaris MBBS BSc MSc FRCS
Director of Transplantation
Consultant Renal and Transplant Surgeon,
St George's Hospital, London

Mr Shahid A. Khan BSc Hons MBBS PhD FRCP
Consultant Gastroenterologist and Hepatologist,
The London Clinic Consulting Rooms, London

Mr Varun R. Kshettry BA
Research Intern, Minneapolis Heart Institute,
Minneapolis, Minnesota

Dr Vibhu R. Kshettry MD FRCS FACS
Director, Cardiovascular and Transplant Surgery,
Minneapolis Heart Institute, Minneapolis, Minnesota

Professor Shaun R. McCann MB FRCPI FRCPEdin FRCPath
Consultant Haematologist, Professor of Haematology,
Department of Haematology
St James Hospital and University of Dublin Trinity College,
Dublin

Mr Madhava Pai MS MSc DIC MRCS (Edin) FRCS (Gen Surg)
Senior Clinical Fellow,
Department of HPB Surgery, Hammersmith Hospital,
London, UK

Mr Vassilios Papalois MD PhD FICS FRCS
Consultant Surgeon, Reader in Transplantation Surgery
The West London Renal and Transplant Centre,
Hammersmith Hospital, London

Mr Chad K. Rostron FRCOphth
Consultant Ophthalmologist,
Moorfields Eye Department,
St George's Hospital, London

Mr Asim Syed MRCS
Transplant Fellow
The West London Renal and Transplant Centre,
Hammersmith Hospital, London

Mr John R. C. Telfer FRCS (Glas)
Consultant Plastic Surgeon,
Canniesburn Plastic Surgery Unit, Glasgow

Professor Anthony N. Warrens DM PhD FHEA FRCP
Professor in Renal Medicine and Immunology,
St. Bartholomew's Hospital, London

Foreword

Much has changed over the last 100 years since the birth of transplantation with the work of Alexis Carel. No one could have ever imagined then that so many different organs could have been so successfully transplanted. At the beginning the question was whether it was ethical to perform a transplant; now, conversely, the ethical dilemma revolves around why a patient should not be transplanted.

The advances in transplantation have revolutionized medicine and surgery and have given us food for thought for many other specialities. Indeed, transplantation is a multidisciplinary speciality with contributors from all fields of medicine.

I am delighted to write this foreword for the second edition of *Introduction to Organ Transplantation*. This volume yields a valuable overview of the tremendous progress made in the recent decades. It starts with a chapter on the history of organ and cell transplantation leading to a chapter on the Ethical issues. A chapter on HLA which was written in the first edition by the father of histocompatibility complex, Jean Dausset, has been updated by his sucessor Jacques Colombani. This is followed by chapters on skin, kidney, pancreas, liver, heart, cornea, small bowel, stem cells, homeostasis in organ donors and a final chapter on recent advances in immunosuppression.

It has been written by experts in their fields and brings a clear update of the current status of transplantation. The overall quality was accomplished through excellent contributions recruited from around the world. It is a good introduction to the field of transplantation for the general reader and undergraduate students with an interest in this field. It will serve as an invaluable resource to anyone interested in a global view of the practice of transplantation.

David Taube
Professor of Transplantation Medicine and Medical Director
Imperial College Healthcare NHS Trust

1

History of Organ and Cell Transplantation*

Nadey S. Hakim and Vassilios Papalois

Over the years, transplantation has fascinated the scientific community as well as the general public for a variety of reasons. The development of transplantation has involved almost all medical specialities. In the history of medicine, perhaps there is no other better example of so extensive a co-operation and exchange of knowledge and experience amongst basic scientists, surgeons and physicians in achieving a common goal.

1.1 HLA and Transplantation Immunology

The classic human skin graft experiments of Gibson and Medawar[1] in 1943 demonstrated the immunologic specificity of allograft rejection — donor specific response, systemic immunity and immunological memory.

Scientific advances in the fields of immunology and genetics provided a fertile environment for the discovery and characterization of the human

---

*This chapter is based on: Hakim, N. and Papalois, V. (eds.) (2003). *History of Organ and Cell Transplantation*, World Scientific Publishing, Singapore.

major histocompatibility complex (MHC; in humans it is the human leuko-cyte antigen: HLA). Today, we know that HLA is a gene complex found in a four-megabase region on the short arm of chromosome 6. Three groups of major histocompatibility complex loci have been described: Class I, Class II and Class III. The first alloantibodies to Class I HLA were identified by Dausset[2,3] and Miescher and Fouconnet[4] in leukaemia patients who had received blood transfusions.

1.1.1 Initial use of cell culture methodologies to detect major histocompatibility complex (MHC) products

In 1964, Bain *et al.*[5] and Bach and Hirschhorn[6] reported that when mix-tures of leukocytes from two unrelated individuals were cultured together for several days, large DNA synthesizing lymphoblasts appeared in the cultures. Bach and Hirschhorn[6] suggested that quantitation of the degree of transfor-mation in these cultures might measure the histocompatibility of recipient–donor combinations. These tests developed into what is now known as the mixed lymphocyte culture (MLC).

The World Health Organization (WHO) committee for HLA nomencla-ture is responsible for naming alleles and periodically publishing an update of new alleles. Regardless of the method used for HLA typing, the challenge continues to be the interpretation of results in light of the available sequence information.

1.1.2 Genomic organization of the HLA complex

The understanding of the HLA complex has been expanded with studies of the protein products and genomic analyses.

1.1.3 Organizations

Particularly beneficial to collaboration among early serologists was the establishment of a serum bank by the National Institute of Allergy and Infectious Diseases (NIAID).[7] The National Institutes of Health (NIH) Serum Bank, housed at the NIH in Bethesda, Maryland, USA, and headed by Don Kayhoe, served as a repository for sera contributed by recipients of NIH contracts specifically designed to procure typing reagents, as well as sera contributed by many other generous investigators. This repository provided start-up reagents to new typing laboratories and reference reagents for national and international workshops. It also supported training workshops for technologists and laboratory directors who were just starting new tissue-typing laboratories.

During the past half-century, knowledge of the structure, function and regulation of the HLA has increased at a rapid rate. Yet, its precise role in allotransplantation remains elusive and controversial. The genetic complexity of the MHC, the incompleteness of our knowledge of it, the great variety of antigens which it presents to the immune system, the interaction of the MHC with a myriad of other immune effector molecules (some of which are encoded by genes closely linked to the MHC Class I and Class II genes) – all of these factors (and more) greatly complicate our ability to fully understand the relative importance of MHC antigen-matching and avoidance of donor-specific anti-HLA antibodies for improving the likelihood of successful allotransplantation.

1.2 Organ Donation and Sharing

1.2.1 The early kidney programmes

The transplantation of the kidney paved the way for the transplantation of other organs. The first human-to-human kidney transplant was from a postmortem donor to a sublimate-intoxicated female. Y.Y. Voronoy performed the operation in 1933 in the Ukraine. In the United States, David Hume started kidney transplantation in 1947, followed by three teams in Paris in 1950. Most of the transplants were cadaveric and for a short time successful, but for no longer than a few weeks. In France, the kidneys of a guillotined criminal were procured right after the execution and divided between two teams in two separate hospitals.

1.2.2 The exchange programmes

In 1967, the first international exchange organization, Eurotransplant, was founded in Western Europe.[8] This exchange programme involved

West Germany, Luxembourg, Belgium and the Netherlands. There was no governmental involvement. The basis of the collaboration was the finding with HLA-typing that a good match gave a better result.

France followed suit in 1969 with the exchange programme Scandia-transplant and United Kingdom and Ireland Renal Transplant Consortium (UKIRTC) was created in 1972. An interstate kidney-sharing programme was established in Australia in the early 1980s.[9]

1.2.3 The donors

The first human kidney transplant with long-lasting success was performed in 1954 in Boston, USA.[10] The crucial point in this case was the fact that donor and recipient were identical twins, proven by skin transplants. The kidney lasted for eight years. The technique was the same as the one developed by the Paris teams in 1950: end-to-side artery and vein to the external iliac vessels and an ureteroneocystomy. This technique has survived until the present day.

1.2.4 Brain death

The concept of *coma dépassé* originated in France and opened the possibility to procure organs for transplantation while the heart is still beating. In 1963, the Belgian surgeon Guy Alexandre was the first to start *coma dépassé*, followed by the team co-ordinated by Hamburger in Paris in 1964.[11]

1.2.5 The nonrenal organs

Successful liver transplantation only became possible when heart-beating donation became a reality and when cyclosporine, a stronger immunosuppressant drug, became available (1980 onwards). When a liver was too large for a small recipient, reduced-sized livers were used.

The heart has a special position in organ donation and sharing — only after the acceptance of the concept of brain death can heart transplantation become possible. Short preservation time restricts sharing and again there is not much to win with matching for the heart transplant as matching does not affect success rate.

1.3 The History of Kidney Transplantation

1.3.1 1902–1912: Experimental efforts of Ullmann and Carrel

At the Vienna Medical Society meeting in January 1902, Hungarian surgeon Emerich Ullmann reported the first case of kidney transplantation, in which a dog's kidney was implanted into another dog's neck.[11,12]

Also in 1902, French surgeon Alexis Carrel, apparently unaware of Ullmann's work, published a paper in the journal *Lyon Médecine* entitled 'The Operating Technique for Vascular Anastomosis and Organ Transplantation'.[13]

In 1904, Carrel left Lyon for the United States. From 1905 to 1906, he worked in Chicago in close collaboration with Charles Guthrie, where the two investigators made significant contributions in the field of vascular grafts and organ transplantation.

1.3.2 1906–1913: Initial kidney transplants from animals to humans

The French surgeon Mathieu Jaboulay was the first to clearly document kidney transplants from animals to humans.[14] In 1906, he transplanted the left kidney of a pig into the left elbow of a woman suffering from nephrotic syndrome. However, this graft failed because of early vascular thrombosis.

1.3.3 1936: First unsuccessful kidney transplant between humans

In 1936, in Kherson, Russia, Voronoy reported the first kidney transplant between humans using a cadaveric kidney.[15] The recipient was a 26-year-old woman who was admitted in a uraemic coma after swallowing mercury in a suicide attempt. Voronoy retrieved a kidney from a 60-year-old man who had died from a fracture of the base of the skull.

1.3.4 1943–1944: Medawar's explanation of graft destruction due to 'biological incompability', as described by Carrel

During World War II, the British Medical Research Council (MRC) focused on the problem of skin grafting for the treatment of burns. They asked Peter Medawar, an Anglo–Lebanese professor of zoology, to work with Thomas Gibson, a plastic surgeon, to attempt to perfect skin auto- and, if possible, allotransplantation in humans.[16] In the laboratory, Medawar observed a persistent finding in experiments with mice or rabbits: if an initial skin graft was taken from animal A and placed on animal B, it survived for about seven days. Then, if a second skin graft was taken from animal A and placed on animal B in exactly the same fashion, it was destroyed in about half that period of time.

Medawar characterized this finding as the 'second set response' and defined its immunologic origin.[17,18] Carrel's description of graft destruction due to 'biological incompatibility' was now explained as rejection due to an immunologic response.

Medawar, in collaboration with Brent and Billingham, proceeded to unravel many aspects of tissue immunology. Medawar's historic achievements established the field of modern transplant immunology, and he shared the Nobel prize in medicine with Sir Frank Macfarlane Burnet in 1960.[18–21]

1.3.5 1947–1953: Initial unsuccessful allotransplants after World War II

In 1947, a young woman was admitted to the Peter Bent Brigham Hospital in Boston, USA. The decision to have her undergo a kidney transplant was made by a team led by David Hume.[22] The hospital administration objected to the use of an operating theatre for such an experimental procedure, so the operation was performed in the middle of the night under difficult conditions, in a small room, using only two lamps.

In 1950, at the Presbyterian Hospital in Chicago, Richard H. Lawler replaced the left kidney of a woman who had a compromised prognosis because of complicated polycystic kidney disease. By six months post-transplant, the graft was completely destroyed. The recipient lived for some time with just her right polycystic kidney.

In January 1951, in Paris, two kidney transplants were performed on the same day by two different teams. Charles Dubost and Nicolaos Oeconomos used a kidney that had been retrieved from a prisoner immediately after his execution by guillotine.[23]

Later that same month, also in Paris, René Küss performed a kidney transplant in a 44-year-old woman with advanced renal failure.[24] This case was most likely the first kidney transplant from a living donor.

1.3.6 1959: First successful kidney transplant between nonidentical twins

In January 1959, the first successful kidney transplant between dizygotic twins was performed, again at the Peter Bent Brigham Hospital in Boston, USA, by a team led by Murray.[25]

1.3.7 1960: First successful kidney transplant between nontwin siblings

In January 1960, the first successful kidney transplant between nontwin siblings took place at the Foch Hospital in Surenes, France, and was performed by a team led by René Küss.[26]

1.3.8 1960–1961: First successful kidney transplant between nonsiblings

In 1960 and 1961, at the Foch Hospital, Küss performed two kidney transplants between nonsiblings. An episode of rejection occurred at five weeks post-transplant. It was treated with low doses of total body irradiation, steroids and, based on the results of the experimental studies conducted by Roy Calne, 6-mercaptopurine, a new agent with a highly immunosuppressive effect in animals.[27]

1.3.9 1961–1962: First kidney transplants using azathioprine

Experimentation with 6-mercaptopurine began in 1959 in London, where Roy Calne demonstrated prolonged kidney graft survival in dogs.[27]

This drug was first used in humans in 1960, as a complement to initial total body irradiation.

1.3.10 1962: First successful cadaveric kidney transplant using immunosuppression

In April 1962, at the Peter Bent Brigham Hospital, Murray performed the first successful human cadaveric kidney transplant, using an immunosuppressive regimen of azathioprine and actinomycin C.[28] The graft functioned for more than one year — a record for a cadaveric kidney at that time.

1.4 The History of Liver Transplantation

In the USA, in the late 1950s and early 1960s, two independent attempts at orthotopic liver transplantation in the dog were made. These were by Dr Francis Moore at the Peter Bent Brigham Hospital in Boston and by Dr Thomas Starzl in the Northwestern University of Chicago.[29,30] As Starzl has pointed out, the Boston group were continuing their interest in organ transplantation following their unique and extensive experience of kidney transplantation, whereas in Chicago Dr Starzl was particularly interested in the metabolism of the liver and especially a comparison of systemic venous blood and portal venous blood entering the liver. A major obstacle in performing the orthotopic operation was the fatal result of clamping the portal vein and inferior vena cava (IVC) in the dog during the recipient hepatectomy.

The early cases of liver transplantation in Denver, where Starzl moved in 1961, proved to be formidable surgical undertakings. By October 1963, the Denver group had had no long-term success and had decided to have a moratorium on orthotopic liver transplantation, which lasted for more than three years. In 1967,[31] the Denver group resumed orthotopic liver transplantation obtaining some long-term successes.

In 1968, Roy Calne achieved the first technically successful liver transplant in Europe.[32] A lady with a primary malignant growth in her liver was referred to Calne. She was anxious to go through this new and experimental operation, even after she had been told the numerous dangers — she said she had nothing to lose. Most of Roy Calne's colleagues at Addenbrooke's Hospital were opposed to him doing a liver graft for a variety of reasons. Then, on 2 May 1968, a child with a viral brain infection became comatose, with irreversible destruction of the brain stem.

Calne convened a meeting of his colleagues to discuss the case. That morning, Francis Moore had phoned him. By extraordinary good fortune, he happened to be in Cambridge visiting his son, a graduate student in molecular biology. Calne asked Moore to join the meeting. When the details of both the recipient and potential donor had been presented, Calne asked each of his colleagues for an opinion. They were unanimous in opposing the operation.

Calne introduced the world-famous Dr Moore, who, together with Starzl, was one of the pioneers in liver grafting. Moore's response was short and typical of him: 'Roy, you have to do it.' Their patient woke up shortly after the end of the operation, and all were delighted. Sadly, two and a half months later, she developed a fatal pneumonia due to the immunosuppressive drugs given to prevent organ rejection.

1.5 Multi-Visceral Transplants

Multi-visceral transplants in which the liver is a component organ have figured experimentally and clinically over the years. With the introduction of cyclosporine there has been a number of attempts at intestinal and liver transplants, when the patient has had liver disease in addition to the need for small bowel replacement.

1.6 The History of Pancreas Transplantation

The idea of pancreas transplantation as a treatment for diabetes has been present ever since the disease was recognized as a deficiency of insulin secretion in the pancreas. In the 1920s, when insulin was isolated and parental administration for treatment of the disease became widespread, vascularization of pancreas allografts was also performed in dogs.[33]

In the next few decades, various investigators worked out some of the surgical details of pancreas transplantation in animal models,[33–40] thus setting the stage for clinical application.[41]

1.6.1 Clinical chronology

The first human pancreas allograft was performed by doctors William D. Kelly and Richard C. Lillihei on 16 December 1966 at the University of Minnesota. The International Pancreas Transplant Registry (IPTR) was formed at the Lyon meeting in 1980.[42,43] The progressive improvement in pancreas transplant outcomes over time has been well documented by the IPTR through annual reports.[44,45] By 2000, more than 15,000 pancreas transplants had been reported to the IPTR (80% from the United States), with more than 1,000 annually since the mid 1990s.

1.6.2 Evolution of recipient selection and programme development

In addition to the observations on secondary complications, studies in the 1980s documented an improvement in the day-to-day quality of life of a diabetic patient by the insulin independence induced by a functioning pancreas graft.[46,47] Follow-up studies confirmed this benefit,[48] providing an impetus to consider pancreas (or islet) transplantation at any stage of diabetes.

1.7 The Development of Islet Transplantation

1.7.1 The first successful islet isolation and transplantation

The transplantation of vascularized organs (such as the kidney) was gaining much attention by the late 1950s, with the phenomenon of allograft rejection documented and under intense investigation. The possibility of transplanting endocrine tissue (parathyroid) as a free graft was first investigated as a scientific endeavour by Russell, who raised the intriguing possibility that such tissue might show reduced immunogenicity.[49] The improved yields of islets obtained using the collagenase digestion technique allowed Moskalewski (working with Hellman in Uppsala, Sweden), to report the first study of survival of transplanted isolated islets.[50] However, the real credit for realizing the full potential of isolated islet transplantation goes to Lacy in St Louis,[51] who took the collagenase digestion technique reported by Moskalewski and combined it with a pre-digestion process of intraductal distension with mechanical mincing of the pancreatic tissue in order to improve the efficiency of the collagenase. Using this technique, Lacy and co-workers[52] were able to obtain sufficient islets to demonstrate an effect on plasma glucose following isologous islet transplantation to the peritoneal cavity of streptozotocin diabetic rats. By today's standards, these first islet transplants showed minimal function, but nevertheless the results were greeted with much excitement.

1.7.2 Development of techniques for identification, tissue culture and cryopreservation of islet tissue, and assessment of islet viability and function

A number of ancillary techniques developed over the years have been important in facilitating advances in islet isolation and transplantation. The ability to easily identify islet tissue *in vitro* is a facility now taken for granted as the use of dithizone allows visualization of islet tissue, causing the zinc-containing islets to stain bright red. The affinity of dithizone for islet tissue was noted many years before it was rediscovered as useful in isolated islet identification.[53,54]

For rapid islet viability assessment, many groups used dye exclusion techniques common to all tissue culture labs, but the use of supravital fluorescent dyes requiring active uptake provided a more accurate definition of viability and was first introduced and validated for islets by Derek Gray from Morris' group in Oxford, UK.[55]

1.7.3 Clinical islet transplantation

The ultimate goal of all the aforementioned experiments has been to successfully transplant islets into diabetic patients, producing as close to a true cure by replacement as it may be possible to get. Early attempts to achieve this goal using tissue obtained from techniques designed for rodent pancreas were uncritical in terms of definition of exactly what was being transplanted, and the results were very poor. Indeed, clinical islet transplantation more or less ceased (ignoring sporadic reports that were not repeatable) until a repeatable technique, which could regularly isolate large numbers of islets from the human pancreas, became available, with the aforementioned advances in automation.

Most reports of successful islet transplantation utilized several donors to obtain sufficient islets in order to obtain insulin independence, and most of the centres took the approach of trying to reduce the number of donors required to one, the Giessen group being the most successful in this aim.[56–59] However, the importance of being able to achieve insulin independence, albeit using multiple organ donors, was highlighted by the extraordinary interest generated from the report by Lakey and Shapiro from Rajotte's group in Edmonton, who obtained insulin independence in seven consecutive patients by using islets from multiple donors, combined with a novel, steroid-sparing immunosuppressive regimen.[60]

1.8 The History of Intestinal Transplantation

1.8.1 The world experience

Between April 1985 and May 2001, 651 patients worldwide received 696 intestinal transplants at 55 centres,[61] 180 (28%) of which were performed at the University of Pittsburgh, USA. The number of centres involved and procedures performed increased each year. The kind of allografts used were isolated intestine (42%), combined liver–intestine (43%), and multi-visceral (14%). In children (61% of the recipients), the underlying diseases were gastroschisis (21%), volvulus (18%), dysmotility syndromes (18%), necrotizing enterocolitis (12%), intestinal atresia (7%) and microvillus inclusion (6%). For adults (39% of total cases), the indications for transplantation were intestinal vascular occlusive disease (22%), Crohn's disease (13%), gastrointestinal neoplasms (13%) and trauma (12%). The retransplantation rate was 7% for children and 5% for adults.

1.8.2 The Pittsburgh experience

At the University of Pittsburgh, a total of 165 transplants were given to 155 consecutive recipients between May 1990 and February 2001. The actuarial patient survival for the total population was 75% at one year, 54% at five years, and 42% at ten years, with achievement of full nutritional autonomy in more than 90% of survivors.[62]

1.8.3 Future prospects

The emergence of intestinal transplantation has depended on the development of more potent immunosuppression, and particularly the advent of tacrolimus. This progress has culminated in the qualification of these procedures for funding as a service by the US's Health Care Financing Administration (HCFA) as of 4 October 2000. The further maturation of the field will almost certainly be contingent on better timing and more discriminating doses of immunosuppressants.

1.9 The History of Heart Transplantation and Heart Valve Transplantation

The possibility of human heart transplantation was first entertained in the early 1900s, starting with a heterotopic heart transplant performed by Alexis Carrel and Charles Guthrie in 1905 at the University of Chicago.[63] Such experiments were performed to establish the techniques of vascular anastomoses. This first reported heart transplant was performed by transplanting a smaller dog heart into the neck of a larger dog. The transplanted heart survived for about two hours.[64]

Orthotopic heart transplantation was first performed by Petrovich Demikhov in the early 1950s. He devised a method of sequential anastomoses to maintain both donor and recipient perfusion during orthotopic heart-lung transplantation without use of cardiopulmonary bypass.[64]

1.9.1 Clinical heart transplantation in humans

The era of clinical human heart transplantation began in 1964 when James D. Hardy, at the University of Mississippi Medical Center, performed a chimpanzee-to-human orthotopic heart transplant.[65] On 3 December 1967, Christian N. Barnard performed the first successful human orthotopic heart transplant at Groote Schuur Hospital in Cape Town, South Africa.[66] The recipient survived for 18 days before succumbing to *Pseudomonas* pneumonia.

1.9.2 Heart valve transplantation

Early heart valve replacements were performed with crude mechanical valves that were highly thrombogenic. This led to the implantation of homografts, first inserted in 1962 by Donald Ross in London and Brian Barrett-Boyes in Auckland.[67,68] In the 1960s and early 1970s, homografts were the biological valve of choice. However, there were difficulties in harvesting as well as limited lifespan of the homograft. This stimulated further research efforts for alternative bioprostheses, paving the way for the introduction of porcine, and later, pericardial bioprosthetic valves.

1.10 Lung Transplantation

The world's first human lung transplant was performed at the University of Mississippi Medical Center by Dr James D. Hardy in 1963. This procedure was performed in a 58-year-old prison inmate who was suffering from chronic infection, abscess and atelectasis formation in his left lung. The patient survived for 18 days and maintained excellent arterial oxygen saturations for the first week post-transplant. Immunosuppressive therapy had not been developed and was not used in this first human lung transplant.

1.10.1 Living-related lobar lung transplantation

The success of human lung transplantation has improved due to advancements in surgical technique, donor organ preservation, prevention and treatment of rejection, and management of infection. This has resulted in an expansion of recipient selection criteria and increased demand for donor organs. Starnes *et al.* have reported the results of eight patients with a variety of diagnoses, including primary pulmonary hypertension, post-chemotherapy, pulmonary fibrosis, bronchopulmonary dysplasia, idiopathic pulmonary fibrosis and obliterative bronchiolitis.[69] Overall survival at one year was 75%. These results support an expanded role for living-donor lobar lung transplantation. Survival at four years post-transplant is approximately 50% for paediatric and adult lung transplant recipients combined. Continuing research efforts, donor and recipient selection and management, and clinical trials using a variety of new immunosuppressive agents will potentially improve the overall results of lung transplantation.

1.11 Bone Marrow Transplantation

1.11.1 Early attempts at BMT

The first published attempt at human bone marrow transplantation was by the doyen and Nobel-prize winner E. Donal Thomas in 1957.[70] Although this attempt was unsuccessful, it did demonstrate that large amounts of marrow could be safely infused intravenously.

1.11.2 The new era

In 1968, the team of Robert Good carried out a bone marrow transplant in Minneapolis based on results of histocompatibility tests in a child with severe immunological deficiency.[69,70]

The major clinical problems are finding histocompatible sibling donors, prevention of graft rejection, support care with blood products, antibodies antivirals and antifungals, prevention and treatment of graft–versus–host disease and veno–venous occlusive disease of the liver and longterm management of gonadal failure and sterility in adults.[69,70]

1.11.3 New developments

To obtain adequate amounts of bone marrow for transplantation, approximately one litre of marrow is removed from the iliac crest of the donor. This is a relatively cumbersome procedure and usually requires general anaesthesia.

1.12 Arm Transplantation

Earl Owen, world-renowned pioneer of microsurgery, first voiced the idea of a hand transplant more than 30 years ago in a speech at Edinburgh University, but it was not until the mid 1990s that he decided it was both technically and immunologically possible. The only reported hand transplant attempt had taken place in Ecuador in 1964 and had failed due to initial absence of any anti-rejection drug use, allowing immediate severe rejection.

With this in mind, and with encouraging results of successful skin, nerve and joint human transplants, he approached Nadey Hakim in 1998, who contacted the Royal College of Surgeons and the UK's Transplant Service Authority to ask for permission for such an operation to go ahead. However, British authorities were unconvinced and had doubts about the ethics of the procedure for a single limb. They believed that putting a healthy patient on potentially dangerous immunosuppressants could not be justified at this stage, despite the long-term successes with experimental animal composite tissue transplants with a cocktail of recently proven powerful drugs.

Owen was keen to form a team of experts in preparation for the procedure, so Hakim suggested that he contact Max Dubernard, head of transplantation and urology at Lyon's Edouard Herriot Hospital. Dubernard had carried out France's first pancreas transplant in 1976 and was not only one of France's top surgeons, but also a prominent local politician who ran his own hospital department. He was excited by Owen's suggestion and agreed that the proposed forearm transplant could go ahead in his department in Lyon. Owen quietly began assembling a skilled international team composed of transplant, orthopaedic and hand microsurgeons, anaesthetists, a psychiatrist and a psychologist specializing in body image disturbances.

A gentleman called Clint Hallam was well known to Owen and was one of three people shortlisted for a hand transplant. Hallam, determined for many years to have the operation, had contacted Owen and confirmed his willingness to travel for the surgery anywhere, anytime.

The surgical team was drawn from around the world and therefore its members needed to agree on a time to convene and then wait for a donor to become available. The date was set for the beginning of September, 1998. The operation went very smoothly, and the team went on to perform the first successful double arm transplant — another global first. The recipient of the new hands, Denis Chatelier, was a 33-year-old house painter and father of two, whose hands were blown off when a home-made model rocket he was showing to his nephews exploded prematurely.

References

1. Gibson, T. and Medawar, P.B. (1943). The Fate of Skin Homografts in Man, *J Anat*, **77**, 299–310.
2. Dausset, J. (1952). Leuco-agglutinins. IV. Leuco-agglutinins and Blood Transfusion, *Vox Sang*, **4**, 190–198.
3. Dausset, J.A. and Nenna, A. (1952). Présence d'une leuco-agglutinine dans le sérum d'un cas d'agranulocytose chronique, *Compt Rend Soc Biol*, **149**, 1539–1541.
4. Miescher, P. and Fauconnet, M. (1954). Mise en évidence de différents groupes leucocytaires chez l'homme, *Schweiz Med Wochenschr*, **84**, 597–599.
5. Bain, B., Vasa, M.R. and Lowenstein, L. (1964). The Development of Large Immature Mononuclear Cells in Mixed Leukocyte Cultures, *Blood*, **23**, 108–116.

6. Bach, F.H. and Hirschhorn, K. (1964). Lymphocyte Interaction: A potential histocompatibility test *in vitro*, *Science NY*, **143**, 813–814.
7. Amos, D.B. (1990). 'HLA-A Mouser's Recollections', in Terasaki, P.I. *et al.* (eds), *History of HLA: Ten Recollections*, UCLA Tissue Typing Laboratory, Los Angeles, p. 61.
8. Rood, J.J. *et al.* (1971). Eurotransplant: An Organisation to Arrive at the Best Possible Results in Kidney Transplantation, *Transplant Proc*, **3**, 933–941.
9. McBride, M. and Chapman, J.R. (1995). An Overview of Transplantation in Australia, *Anaesth Intens Care*, **23**, 60–64.
10. Murray, J.E., Merrill, J.P. and Harrison, J.H. (1955). Renal Homotransplantations in Identical Twins, *Surg Forum*, **6**, 432–436.
11. Küss, R. and Bourget, P. (1992). *Une histoire illustrée de la greffe d'organes*, Laboratoire Sandoz, Rueil-Malmaison, France.
12. Peer, L.A. (1955). *Transplantation of Tissues*, Williams and Wilkins, Baltimore, USA, pp. 25–29.
13. Carrel, A. (1902). La technique opératoire des anastomoses vasculaires et la transplantation des viscères, *Lyon Med*, **98**, 859–864.
14. Jaboulay, M. (1906). Greffe de reins au pli du coude par soudures arterielles et veincuses, *Lyon Med*, **107**, 575–577.
15. Voronoy, Y. (1936). Sobre el bloqueo del aparato reticulocndotclial del hombre en algunas formas de intoxicacion por el sublimado y sobre la transplantacion del rinon cadaverico como metodo de lo anuria consecutiva aquella intoxicacion, *Siglo Medico*, **97**, 296–298.
16. Gibson, T. and Medawar, P.B. (1943). The Behaviour of Skin Homografts in Man, *J Anat*, **77**, 299–310.
17. Medawar, P.B. (1944). The Behaviour and Fate of Skin Homografts in Rabbits, *J Anat*, **78**, 176–199.
18. Mcdawar, P.B. (1945). Second Study of Behaviour of Skin Homografts in Rabbits, *J Anat*, **79**, 157–176.
19. Billingham, R.E., Krohn, P.I. and Medawar, P.B. (1951). Effect of Cortisone on Survival of Skin Homografts in Rabbits, *Br Med J*, **1**, 1157–1163.
20. Billingham, R.E., Brent, L. and Medawar, P.B. (1953). Actively Acquired Tolerance of Foreign Cells, *Nature*, **172**, 603–606.
21. Billingham, R.E., Brent, L. and Medawar, P.B. (1956). Quantitative Studies on Tissue Transplantation Immunity. III. Actively Acquired Tolerance, *Philos Trans Roy Soc London Biol Sci*, **239**, 357–412.
22. Hume, D.M. *et al.* (1955). Experiences with Renal Homotransplantations in the Human: Report of Nine Cases, *J Clin Invest*, **34**, 327–382.
23. Dubost, C. *et al.* (1951). Résultats d'une tentative greffe rénale, *Bull Soc Med Hop Paris*, **67**, 1372–1382.
24. Küss, R., Teinturier, J. and Millieaz, P. (1951). Quelques essais de greffe rein chez l'homme, *Meme Acad Chir*, **77**, 754–764.

25. Merrill, J.P. *et al.* (1960). Successful Homotransplantations of the Human Kidney Between Nonidentical Twins, *New Engl J Med*, **262**, 1251–1260.
26. Küss, R. *et al.* (1962). Homologous Human Kidney Transplantation: Experience with Six Patients, *Postgrad Med J*, **38**, 528–531.
27. Calne, R.Y. (1960). The Rejection of Renal Homografts: Inhibition in Dogs by 6-mercaptopurine, *Lancet*, **1**, 417–418.
28. Murray, J.E. *et al.* (1963). Prolonged Survival of Human Kidney Homografts by Immunosuppressive Drug Therapy, *New Engl J Med*, **268**, 1315–1323.
29. Moore, F.D. *et al.* (1959). One-stage Homotransplantations of the Liver Following Total Hepatectomy in Dogs, *Transpl Bull*, **6**, 103–110.
30. Starzl, T.E., Bernhard, V.M., Benvenuto, R. *et al.* (1959). A New Method for One-Stage Hepatectomy in Dogs, *Surgery*, **46**, 880–886.
31. Starzl, T.E. *et al.* (1968). Orthotopic Homotransplantation of the Human Liver, *Ann Surg*, **168**, 392–415.
32. Calne, R.Y. and Williams, R. (1968). Liver Transplantation in Man. I. Observations on Technique and Organisation in Five Cases, *Br Med J*, **4**, 535–550.
33. Gayet, R.C. and Guillamie, M. (1927). La regulation de la secretion interne pancreatique par un processus humoral, demonstree par des transplantations de pancreas. Experiences sue des animaux normaux, *C R Soc Biol*, **97**, 1613–1614.
34. Brooks, J.R. and Gifford, G.H. (1959). Pancreatic Homotransplantations, *Transpl Bull*, **6**, 100–103.
35. De Jode, L.R. and Howard, J.M. (1962). Study in Pancreaticoduodenal Homotransplantation, *Surg Gynecol Obstet*, **114**, 553–558.
36. Bergan, J., Hoehn, J.G. and Porter, N. (1965). Total Pancreatic Allografts in Pancreatectomized Dogs, *Arch Surg*, **90**, 521–526.
37. Largiader, F. *et al.* (1967). Orthotopic Allotransplantation of the Pancreas, *Am J Surg*, **113**, 70–78.
38. Merkel, F.K. *et al.* (1968). Irradiated Hetertopic Segmental Canine Pancreatic Allografts, *Surgery*, **63**, 291–297.
39. Idezuki, Y. *et al.* (1968). Experimental Pancreaticoduodenal Preservation and Transplantation, *Surg Gynecol Obstet*, **126**, 1002–1014.
40. Sutherland, D.E.R. (1981). Pancreas and Islet Transplantation. I. Experimental Studies, *Diabetologia*, **20**,161–185.
41. Lillehei, R.C. *et al.* (1970). Pancreaticoduodenal Allotransplantation: Experimental and Clinical Experience, *Ann Surg*, **172**, 405–436.
42. Dubernard, J.M. and Traeger, J. (1980). Pancreas and Islet Transplantation Workshop, *Transplant Proc*, **12**, 1–2.
43. Sutherland, D.E.R. (1980). International Human Pancreas and Islet Transplant Registry, *Transplant Proc*, **12(4)(Suppl. 2)**, 229–236.
44. Gruessner, A. and Sutherland, D.E.R. (2000). 'Analyses of Pancreas Transplant Outcomes for United States Cases Reported to the United Network for

Organ Sharing (UNOS) and Non-US Cases Reported to the International Pancreas Transplant Registry', in Cecka, J.M. and Terasaki, P.I. (eds.), *Clinical Transplant — 1999*, UCLA Immunogenetics Center, Los Angeles, pp. 51–69.

45. Sutherland, D.E.R. and Moudry, K.C. (1987). Pancreas Transplant Registry: History and Analysis of Cases 1966 to October 1986, *Pancreas*, **2**, 473–488.

46. Nakache, R., Tyden, G. and Groth, C.G. (1989). Quality of Life in Diabetic Patients After Combined Pancreas-Kidney or Kidney Transplantation, *Diabetes*, **38(Suppl. 1)**, 40–42.

47. Zehrer, C.L. and Gross, C.R. (1991). Quality of Life of Pancreas Transplant Recipients, *Diabetologia*, **34(Suppl. 1)**, S145–S149.

48. Nakache, R., Tyden, G. and Groth, C.G. (1994). Long-term Quality of Life in Diabetic Patients After Combined Pancreas-Kidney Transplantation or Kidney Transplantation, *Transplant Proc*, **26**, 510–511.

49. Russell, P.S. and Gittes, R.E. (1959). Parathyroid Transplants in Rats — A Comparison of Their Survival Time With That of Skin Grafts, *J Exp Med*, **109**, 571–588.

50. Moskalewski, S. (1970). 'Comparison of Cultured and Transplanted Islets of the Guinea Pig', in Hellman, B. and Taljedal, I. (eds.), *The Structure and Metabolism of the Pancreatic Islets: A Centennial of Paul Langerhans*, Pergamon Press, Oxford, pp. 69–72.

51. Lacy, P.E. and Kostianovsky, M. (1967). Method for the Isolation of Intact Islets of Langerhams from the Rat Pancreas, *Diabetes*, **16**, 35–39.

52. Ballinger, W.F. and Lacy, P.E. (1972). Transplantation of Intact Pancreatic Islets in Rats, *Surgery*, **72**, 175–186.

53. McNary, W.F. (1954). Zinc-Dithizone Reaction of Pancreatic Islets, *J Histochem Cytochem*, **2**, 185–193.

54. Maske, H. (1957). Interaction Between Insulin and Zinc in the Islets of Langerhans, *Diabetes*, **6**, 335–341.

55. Gray, D.W. and Morris, P.J. (1987). The Use of Fluorescein Diacetate and Ethidium Bromide as a Viability Stain for Isolated Islets of Langerhans, *Stain Technol*, **62**, 373–381.

56. Bretzel, R.G. *et al.* (1999). Improved Survival of Intraportal Pancreatic Islet Cell Allografts in Patients' Type-1 Diabetes Mellitus by Refined Peritransplant Management, *J Mol Med*, **77**, 140–143.

57. Mering, J.V. and Minkowski, O. (1980). Diabetes mellitus nach Pankreas-exstirpation, *Arch Exp Pathol Pharmaco*, **26**, 371–387.

58. Minkowski, O. (1892). Weitere Mittheilungen über den diabetes mellitus nach exstirpation des Pankreas, *Berlin Klin Wochenschr*, **5**, 90–94.

59. Bensley, R.R. (1911). Studies on the Pancreas of the Guinea Pig, *Am J Anat*, **43**, 81–94.

60. Shapiro, A.M. *et al.* (2000). Islet Transplantation in Seven Patients with Type-1 Diabetes Mellitus Using a Glucocorticoid-Free Immunosuppressive Regimen, *N Engl J Med*, **343**, 230–238.

61. Grant, D. (2001). Report of the International Intestinal Transplant Registry, *7th International Small Bowel Transplant Symposium*, September 12–15, Stockholm.

62. Abu-Elmagd, K. *et al.* (2001). Clinical Intestinal Transportation: A Decade of a Single-Center Experience, *Ann Surg*, **234**, 404–417.

63. Carrel, A. and Guthrie, C.C. (1905). The Transplantation of Veins and Organs, *Am Med*, **10**, 1101–1102.

64. Demikhov, V.P. (1962). *Experimental Transplantation of Vital Organs*, Consultants' Bureau, New York, USA.

65. Hardy, J.D. *et al.* (1964). Heart Transplantation in Man, *JAMA*, **188**, 114–122.

66. Barnard, C.N. (1967). A Human Cardiac Transplant: An Interim Report of a Successful Operation Performed at Groote Schuur Hospital, Cape Town, *S Afr Med J*, **41**, 1271–1274.

67. Ross, D.N. (1962). Homograft Replacement of the Aortic Valve, *Lancet*, **2**, 487.

68. Barratt-Boyes, B.G. (1964). Homograft Aortic Valve Replacement in Aortic Incompetence and Stenosis, *Thorax*, **19**, 131–135.

69. Starnes, V.A. *et al.* (1997). Experience with Living Donor Transplantation for Indications Other Than Cystic Fibrosis, *J Thorac Cardiovasc Surg*, **114**, 917–922.

70. Thomas, E.D. *et al.* (1957). Intravenous Infusion of Bone Marrow in Patients Receiving Radiation and Chemotherapy, *N Engl Med*, **257**, 491–496.

2

Ethical Issues in Transplantation

Miran Epstein

Transplant medicine is a huge ethical minefield. Virtually each and every one of its evolving aspects was at some point subject to a heated controversy. For more than five decades now it has challenged our conceptions of identity, personhood, autonomy, death and the body. It has even called into question our time-honoured relations of solidarity, altruism and love. And yet nothing in this field is philosophically challenging in itself. The only thing that accounts for its conceptual and ethical flammability is the enormous bearing it has on some of the most sensitive interests of so many social stakeholders.

This chapter expounds a systematic overview of the major ethical issues surrounding transplantation. It thus highlights the problems, the competing solutions, and the justifications for the latter. However, unlike similar overviews, it does not confine the discussion to the philosophical sphere alone, but draws attention to its social roots too. Let there be no mistake: a philosophical discourse about transplant ethics can certainly yield some interesting insights. However, it would be found seriously wanting if it were to be abstracted from its very own political economy, that is to say, the particular ecology of stakeholders, interests and power relations from which it has emerged and evolved as such.

The benefits of discussing ethical ideas in their constitutive context are too important to pass up. This approach has a unique explanatory power: it can account for the emergence, the specificity, and the social status of such ideas. It also has an acute explicatory power: it can shed new, possibly counterintuitive, light on their social role. Its critical power is particularly valuable: it requires us to not only consider the philosophical justifications of the ethical ideas, but also to question the morality of their very own political economy, a thing they would not normally do. These merits can be demonstrated, for example, on the argument supporting a market in organs (the pro-market argument) even without explicating it at all (a detailed discussion of the argument will be expounded later in this chapter).

Let us first consider the very emergence of the argument and its specificity. Could these be explained by the argument itself? No. Being philosophical in essence, the argument deals with justification, not explanations. Besides, it is the very thing to be explained. Can the social status of the argument be attributed to its veracity or falsity? Again, no. One cannot explain something that is changing, social status in this case, by something that is supposed to be immutable (veracity or falsity). Moreover, the social status of the criterion of veracity or falsity is subject to changes too, and thus becomes part of the object to be explained. A strictly philosophical argument cannot account for its own emergence, specificity, or social status.

The Darwinian metaphor can perhaps help us out here. This model has suggested that a biological mutation is a product of a particular ecology, and that its fate as such depends on its reciprocal interaction with the latter. The same, *mutatis mutandis*, could apply in the case of 'ideic mutations', that is to say, ideas that are generated by society and then compete with each other for social status. The key to their specificity and social status can only be found in their interaction with their constitutive environment. The emergence, the specificity, and the social status of the pro-market argument could thus be understood only in light of the social interests in a market in organs and the circumstances that have bred these interests.

Now let us try to identify the *role* of the pro-market argument, that is to say, its reciprocal effect on the stakeholders. The argument purports to be in the interest of all stakeholders. This is implicit in its claim that its very own object — a market in organs — is in the interest of all stakeholders.

Indeed, if a market in organs complies with some common interest, which is true as each stakeholder has some interest in a market in organs, then this must apply to its supportive argument too. But should we take all that at face value? Not necessarily.

The common interest in a market in organs, hence in its supportive argument, has a history that rests on a certain ecology of social interests, which, as we shall see, reveals a different picture. This ecology shows that buyers and vendors of organs, the main stakeholders who are supposed to benefit from a market in organs, would not have embraced the pro-market argument, let alone the market itself, if they had had more appealing alternatives. Moreover, it also shows that the absence of such alternatives has been caused by other stakeholders who typically happen to have some interest in organ commercialism. This means that the common interest in a market in organs and in its supportive argument is a historical product of power relations. The market and the pro-market argument thus transpire to be doing more than they purport to be doing; while both appeal to a common interest as they say they do, they also conceal and thereby reaffirm the underlying power relations. This conclusion has a potentially disturbing and certainly counterintuitive implication; if we deem the appeal of the pro-market argument to some common interest to be ethical, but also believe the coercion that has generated that interest to be immoral, then we are bound to regard the pro-market argument as the ethics of the immoral. Conclusions of such kind are not just intellectually intriguing — they may have a critical implication as well.

Indeed, the last and by far the most important value of the suggested methodology is its potentially critical implication. Normally, ethical arguments, the pro-market argument included, deal with the morality of a certain solution to some problem. The methodology suggested here requires that we also question the morality of the circumstances that have created the problem and made us form and embrace a particular solution, rather than any other. For if the argument has indeed gained increasing popularity under coercive circumstances, then any attempt to criticize it could make sense only if it addressed those circumstances too. Indeed, the demand to ban commerce in organs would make little sense, and would most likely fail, if it did not also call for a ban on the social conditions that make such commerce so appealing in the first place.

Before we embark on this venture, however, some issues of terminology, scope and classification need to be clarified. Strictly speaking, the term 'transplantation' refers to a surgical intervention whereby solid tissue is removed from a biological source and subsequently implanted in a biological recipient. It differs from both 'implantation', where the source is strictly synthetic, and 'transfusion' — transplantation of nonsolid tissue from a biological source, which is not an essentially surgical intervention.

Ideally, our discussion should cover ethical issues in transplantation, implantation and transfusion, as these practices share many of their ethical issues. This book is about surgery, however. For this technical reason we shall have to confine the discussion to issues that involve transplantation and implantation only. Some attention will be given to issues involving prosthetic (artificial) and xenogeneic (animal) grafts. However, the better part of the discussion will be dedicated to the most contentious issues — those that involve organs from human sources.

How the ethical issues are to be sorted is another matter. Some overviews group them as donor-related versus recipient-related. This may be somewhat misleading, however, since the issues invariably involve and affect other stakeholders as well. Besides, implantation, for example, involves no donor at all, hence has no donor issues. An alternative categorization that drew on the specific nature of the different grafts could make sense; however, it would run the risk of obscuring the general themes. To tackle these concerns, we shall classify the issues according to the general practical contexts in which they arise (procurement of organs versus their distribution) and the general source of the graft to which they pertain (artificial, animal, human).

2.1 The Political Economy of Transplantation

A spectre is haunting transplant medicine, the spectre of the 'organ crisis'. Referring to a disturbing gap between demand and supply, this crisis seems to be getting worse. The USA, for example, saw a 46% increase in the absolute number of donors between 1995 and 2008, but the patient-to-donor ratio has increased at a much faster rate (142%) and continues to grow. In 2009, the number of patients with end-stage renal disease (ESRD) listed for transplantation stood at just over 77,000 with only 16,000 receiving transplantation in that year. Another 25,000 patients were waiting for other organs, mainly heart, lung, liver and pancreas.[1] The British experience is essentially similar. In March 2008, 7,500 patients were on the active transplant lists, and a further 2,000 were on the temporarily suspended transplant lists. This represents an increase of 6% and 10%, respectively, compared to the corresponding figures from the previous year.[2] The trend in Europe is somewhat different with a slight drop in the patient-to-donor ratio, but the number of patients on the waiting list saw a thirtyfold increase from 1969 to 2006.

The transplant discourse purports to account for the origins of this crisis by putting the blame on morbidity rates increasing faster than procurement rates. Albeit true, this explanation is not really informative. As a matter of fact, it is the very thing to be explained. A satisfactory explanation requires uncovering the conditions and the circumstances that have bred these trends. These should concern us here not so much because they can explain the evolution of the organ crisis, but rather because they happen to hold the key to understanding why its satellite ethical discourse looks as it does. Put differently, the political economy that has given rise to the problem and the political economy that has given rise to its competing solutions are one and the same.

2.1.1 The demand for organs

Like a demand for any other object, the demand for organs is a historical function of the technological ability to utilize them and the social interests in utilizing them (abilities and interests are historically interdependent: each is a product of preceding abilities and interests). Three general interests can be identified in this respect: interests in the technology of transplantation, interests in organs and transplantations, and interests in practices that create a demand for organs. The latter interests dominate the political economy of the demand.

The following sociological map is an abstraction: each stakeholder is described here as the holder of typical interests only. In reality, however, an individual stakeholder may have several interests, of which some may be in conflict with others. For example, a particular person may benefit and suffer from organ failure at the same time. The reader should bear this in mind and thus focus not on how individuals interact, but rather on how the different kinds of interests interact.

When speaking about the demand for organs in general, the interests that first come to mind are those of patients, organ donors and doctors. Each has a different interest in treating organ failure. However, they have developed their individual interests secondary and subject to their failure to satisfy a more basic interest: avoiding or preventing the underlying morbidity in the first place. We often reduce the explanation of this failure to some biological pathophysiology. For example, we attribute the rising incidence of ESRD and end-stage liver disease (ESLD) to obesity, diabetes and alcoholic liver cirrhosis. This is the truth, of course, but not the whole truth. These conditions have a social *pathophysiology* as well. Indeed, they are largely inflicted by certain forms of production and consumption, which are typically driven by profit. The political economy of the crisis would not be complete without mentioning the financial interests in such practices. As we shall see, the power relations between the beneficiaries of these practices and their victims have been reaffirmed by the ethical discourse: suggestions to manage the crisis have predominated in the discourse, while demands to eradicate its basic causes have been marginalized.

Some other players who have an interest in organs are driven by profit or funding, depending on whether the system in question is private or public, respectively. This group includes the hosting medical institution, the transplant system, its supporting technological and pharmaceutical industries, and, under certain circumstances, even organ brokers and the travel and tourism business.

Payers and purchasers of health care — states, insurers, providers and taxpayers – are interested in organ transplants for their cost-saving effect. Their demand for organs tends to be selective, however, as some transplants are cost-effective compared to the alternatives, whereas others may not be cost effective at all. Kidney transplant, for example, has the biggest cost-saving capacity, considering the relatively large number of patients with renal failure and the high cost of dialysis per patient. Although its cost per patient (around £ 46,000) is more than the annual cost of dialysis (around £ 25,000), once the transplantation has been done, annual treatment expenses drop to £ 7,000 each year, a saving of £ 18,000 per patient per annum. The overall saving is more than double, however. Thus every

2,400 kidney transplantations done in a certain year would save the payer a total of one billion pounds over the next decade.[3-5]

The cost-saving capacity of certain organ transplants is obviously compatible with the profit-maximizing interest of private sector payers, e.g. private health-care insurers. The case of public-sector payers is different, though. Their need to control expenses is not essential to their nature. It has been imposed on them under certain historical circumstances. A comprehensive discussion of this point exceeds the scope of this chapter. However, suffice it to mention that the general funding problem of the public-sector payer has not been caused by any objective scarcity. On the contrary, it is the effect of unequal distribution and redistribution of social wealth that takes place within a rather affluent society. Here too, the domination of the interests of the beneficiaries of that system has been reaffirmed by the ethical discourse; suggestions to manage the crisis have predominated in the discourse, while demands to eradicate its basic causes have been marginalized.

2.1.2 The supply of organs

The supply of organs has a political economy too. Some of the factors are already familiar to us, since they also play a role in the formation of the demand. In general, the pertinent vectors either enhance or hamper the supply, but some of them happen to have a double effect. The fact that there is some supply at all implies that the positive effect outweighs the negative one. However, this does not necessarily entail that the supply meets the demand. The very reality of the organ crisis implies rather the opposite.

Social conditions that breed solidarity and hence interests in mutual aid tend to increase organ donation. Religious and other cultural beliefs may play a positive role in this respect. Occasionally, they rather limit the supply. Some communities of Jewish Orthodox conviction, for example, forbid both deceased and living organ donation, but not reception.[6] In other societies, reluctance to sign a donor card or donate organs of deceased relatives may be secondary to cultural reluctance to receive cadaveric organs. Misunderstanding of the way death is established, distrust in the motivations of the medical authorities, and perhaps even awareness of the inferiority of cadaveric organs relative to organs from the living, are negative factors as well. In addition, reluctance to sign a donor card is commonly attributed to laziness, indifference and unawareness. These phenomena are known to thrive in the absence of effective donor recruitment programmes. Indeed, the efficiency of such programmes has a direct bearing on the supply of organs.

The general social interest in protecting life may paradoxically limit the supply of organs. The legal ban on harvesting hearts from living donors demonstrates this point very well, and so does the drop in the rates of road traffic accidents. On the other hand, the very demand for hearts in itself has had a positive effect on their supply in a way that is arguably less concerned with protecting life. It has made an increasingly inclusive definition of death socially palatable. Hearts (and other organs) can now be harvested under circumstances that had been deemed unacceptable until not so long ago. As we shall see, both the formation and the reception of a broad definition of death have had little to do with its philosophical justifiability (although it may well be justified) and everything to do with its usefulness for the stakeholders. We shall also see that certain economic interests primarily drove this trend.

In fact, economic interests also play an important role in the political economy of the supply of organs. The following case is a rather subtle expression of this point. International data indicate that men are less likely to become organ donors and more likely to become recipients than their wives. Our intuition tends to attribute this gender bias to male chauvinism. However, this is an idealistic, and at any rate simplistic, explanation. It also fails to account for the fact that the phenomenon is more striking in poor communities. The different historical positions of men and women vis-à-vis the labour-power market are the fundamental factors in this case. In giving rise to the distorted conception that unpaid labour power has no value whatsoever, they normalize the idea among men and women alike that housewives ought to sacrifice their organs for their needy husbands.[7] Male chauvinism, which transpires to be an ideological epiphenomenon of these relations, may play a mediating role at best.

The profit drive, which has been shown to play an important role in the political economy of the demand for organs, also plays an impor-tant role in their supply. Its impact is complex, however: other factors ignored, it decreases supply from certain sources, but increases it from others.

This double effect is mediated through an increasingly intensifying global economic competition in ways that are described in the following:

(1) A shift of interests.

Extreme economic competition is inclined to replace social solidarity with individualism. It transforms the social circumstances from such where the happiness of the individual depends on the happiness of others to such where the happiness of others becomes an obstacle to one's own happiness. One of the effects of this trend is a decline in the willingness to donate organs. Moreover, the competition also tends to force the competitors to reduce the value of any object they possess, the body included, to exchange value (a trend called 'commodification') and all relations they have with each other to market relations (a trend called 'commercialization'). This has an additional negative effect on the willingness to donate. Once a price tag has been attached to an object that had previously been given free of charge, a kidney, for example, the general willingness to donate it will tend to erode independently of the underlying commodification process.

The resulting shift from altruistic interests and relations of gift to egoistic interests and relations of commodity probably affects rich and poor equally, but its impact on the organ question generally varies according to the economic status of the player: the poor are more likely to sell their organs than the rich, the rich are more likely to buy organs than the poor, and both are less likely to donate them free of charge. All in all, this explains very well why ideas that support commerce in organs gain increasing popularity within the ethical discourse.

The specific effect of this shift on the actual supply of organs might be hard to assess, since the prevailing ethico-legal position that still rejects commerce in organs makes it difficult for the new motivations to express themselves freely. As a result, the increasing reluctance to donate organs may not be offset by the corresponding increase in the willingness to sell them. Moreover, such a problem may exist even in a system that allows commerce in organs. Those who can buy organs are unlikely to suffer from any shortage. However, those who cannot are likely to suffer even more because of the negative effect of the system on the willingness to donate organs free of charge. The phenomenon of 'transplant tourism' — patients travelling from one country in which commerce in organs is effectively banned to another country where organs are commercially available — demonstrates a similar problem on a global scale. In decimating the rate of donations in both countries, it has created a problem for both noncommercial albeit funding-dependent transplant centres as well as patients who cannot afford to buy the organs.[8]

(2) Increase in poverty.

Contrary to a common view, contemporary poverty is not a result of idleness or bad luck. Rather, it is a historical outcome of an increasingly unequal distribution and redistribution of resource, power and opportunity, which has been brought about first and foremost by the profit interest. Intriguingly, this interest retains its compensatory potential for any drop in the supply of organs it might have caused also through its active impoverishing effect. As already suggested, the poor, more than anyone else, are likely to consider organ vending as a viable option. Increase in both the rate of poverty as well as its intensity is thus likely to augment the supply of commercial organs, all other things ignored.

(3) Decreased investments in donor programmes.

In giving rise to the cost-containing interest of governments, the economic competition may foster their reluctance to invest in donor programmes with a concomitant drop in donation rates. The new Israeli Transplant Law, for example, introduces financial incentives for donors, but fails to secure a budget to support donor programmes as previously proposed.[9] True, this apparent irrationality could be explained away by showing that the cost-effectiveness of the existing allocation of funding is greater than that of any other alternative, but an empirical support to this effect is still pending.

2.2 Two Great Solutions

We have seen that the organ crisis has been caused by its very own victim. Unsurprisingly, that victim — society — also seeks to resolve it. It has come up with two kinds of solutions: nonconsensual and consensual. Virtually each and every one of the nonconsensual solutions was defended at some point for being moral, and virtually each and every one of the consensual solutions was attacked at some point for being immoral. Since we have no Archimedean criterion of morality, the question cannot be decided philosophically. That said, it is decided socially: we may or may not embrace the 'really' moral solution, but we universally regard the solution that we embrace as 'really' moral, and brand the one that we reject as 'really' immoral. Whether or not there is any moral difference between these categories is thus debatable. That said, there is a discernible sociological difference between them.

Nonconsensual solutions do not conceal their partiality. They neither satisfy, nor do they purport to satisfy, any common interest. On the contrary, they blatantly serve some stakeholders at the expense of others. Solutions of that sort reflect some extreme imbalance of power, either real or desired. Accordingly, they are either imposed by overwhelmingly powerful stakeholders or proposed by weak stakeholders who would like to be overwhelmingly powerful. Examples of the former case include procurement of organs using various forms of violence against their original owners, whereas proposals to ban certain morbidity-inflicting forms of production and consumption are examples of the latter case. It is apparently easier to rob the organs of the have-nots, then to impinge on the property rights of the haves.

In contrast, consensual solutions serve some common interest, that is, an abstract interest that is compatible with some concrete interest of each stakeholder. The debate about a market in organs, for example, demonstrates that consensual solutions can be in conflict with each other. Indeed, the pro-market argument and the anti-market argument are both consensual (or nearly consensual) solutions to the organ crisis. Each appeals to some common interest, albeit a different one.

Consensual solutions present a potential problem, however. In serving some common interest, they tend to give the impression that they serve each and every interest of each and every stakeholder. This is certainly possible, but only if the pertinent political economy is made of agonistic interests only, that is to say, interests that are compatible, or at least not incompatible, with each other. The consensus around the Euclidian geometrical axioms, for example, has so far rested on such a tranquil political economy.[10]

In contrast, the political economy of transplantation is stormy: it contains both agonistic and antagonistic interests, the latter referring to conflicting interests. For example, the interest of the patient in avoiding organ failure is in conflict with any financial interests in organ failure or practices that tend to generate organ failure. In fact, the increase in morbidity rates reflects the dominance of the latter over the former. And yet neither the conflict of the interests nor the domination of some interests on others precludes the emergence of a common interest in organ transplants. On the contrary, they become its parents. Consensual solutions, so it appears, are possible even under coercive circumstances. They simply become hegemonic in that they address a common interest that has effectively been tailored by a dominant stakeholder to suit his own interests.[11]

This point is worth remembering, as the ethical discourse about transplantation is almost entirely made of consensual solutions of the hegemonic type. The very fact that it embraces ideas that purport to increase the organ pool while marginalizing those that suggest ways of reducing the need for organs in the first place is its hallmark. The discourse is conservative, then. Instead of challenging the political economy that generates the crisis, it is largely concerned with where to draw the ethical line insofar as the procurement of organs is concerned. Moreover, as the crisis deepens, it is increasingly inclined to push that line to places that had previously been deemed utterly immoral.

2.3 The Ethical Discourse: Procurement of Organs

2.3.1 Prosthetic implants

Since whole, functioning, prosthetic organs are yet to be developed, the impact of this source on the organ crisis is still marginal. At any rate, the ethical discourse finds only the distribution of prosthetic implants potentially problematic (problems pertaining to their distribution will be discussed later on).[12] In fact, it finds few problems (if any) in their production. This is not surprising, considering the fact that synthetic materials such as metal, plastic or ceramic, which are meant to replace lost tissue, involve no donor and hence no donor issues. Nevertheless, even the production of inanimate objects may raise some ethical issues.

One of these rather marginalized issues concerns the justifiability of producing implants of low cost-effectiveness or clinical efficacy relative to available alternatives. Mechanical bridging devices such as total artificial heart and left ventricular assist devices are good examples. Both their cost-effectiveness and their clinical efficacy are considerably low compared to hearts from human sources. The argument supporting such production appeals to the low and at any rate decreasing supply of transplantable hearts. It also reminds us that these devices purport to provide a temporary solution only until a suitable human equivalent is found. This makes sense.

In contrast, the argument that appeals solely to the 'demand' or 'the autonomous will of the customer' is problematic (interestingly, arguments in support of any commodity rarely appeal to the financial interest of the entrepreneur). If given the choice, autonomous customers would never prefer an inferior product to a superior one. A desire for an inferior product would necessarily imply diminished autonomy. Accordingly, the production and marketing of inferior products could be criticized for being necessarily manipulative.

A closely related issue concerns the nature of the need for certain implants, typically cosmetic implants and such that provide some enhanced function that goes beyond the normal. Here, the implants may not be inferior to any alternative. As a matter of fact, they are unlikely to have any equivalent alternative at all. Nonetheless, a need for such implants may have been induced and nurtured by a manipulative industry for the sake of its own profits. An industry that responds to autonomous needs of people is moral, whereas the one that implants heteronomous needs in their minds is not.[13]

2.3.2 **Xenogeneic organs**

The potential benefits of a successful xenograft programme appear to be considerable. The supply of xenografts would in theory be unlimited. The organs could be tailored to the patient's needs. The transplantation could be performed as an elective procedure with therefore better preparation of the patient. There would also be more time to test the animal donor for potential infections compared to the current situation with human transplants. That said, the scientific–technological obstacles to clinical xeno-transplantation are still considerable, and, like prosthetic implants, this source of organs has so far had little if any effect on the crisis. Nevertheless, the ethical discourse was quick to identify its potential problems. Distribution and recipient issues will be discussed later on, but some of them need to be mentioned here, for they have bearing on the ethics of the preliminary scientific work that aims at making this source usable in the first place.

The pertinent issues are two: immunological hurdles and the risk of rejection, and the possible presence of already known and yet undiscovered animal viruses that may put individuals and populations at risk of serious infection.

2.3.2.1 *Clinical trials involving human research subjects*

Against the backdrop of these risks, the first ethical question is not whether it is moral to implant animal organs into humans (so long as the treatment is not viable, the answer is no), but rather whether it is moral to proceed with research, particularly clinical trials, into xenotransplantation.

Typically, the answer is positive. It draws on the argument that success in xenotransplantation would be the best hope for saving the lives of patients with end-stage organ disease, so that the importance of the research objective outweighs the potential risks, which are anyway speculative. Those who are not convinced are seen as fearmongers, blind to the benefits of technology and to human suffering.

This argument raises several objections. First, xenotransplants are currently not the best way to save lives. Transplantation of organs from human sources is available and is known to be relatively safer. Second, it is not justifiable to put individual patients at risk for some uncertain future benefit for other patients. Third, there is evidence that such trials have been driven by money, not by the needs of patients, and that this drive has distorted the scientific information deduced from such trials. In view of these points, it would be impossible to obtain adequately informed consent from research candidates. Moreover, given the fact that the research subjects were all desperately ill, and all transplants resulted in the death of the patients, this question needs to be raised about the past as well. Since the resolution of the ethical and scientific obstacles to xenotransplantation is not guaranteed, one may argue that resources now being directed to it would be better deployed elsewhere.[14]

2.3.2.2 *The use or abuse of animals*

Another set of ethical questions that is not really unique to the issue of xenotransplantation refers to the use of animals in the present research phase and as a future source of tissues and organs.

The first question is about the morality of sacrificing one organism for the sake of another. The question, as it is put, presupposes the possibility that all organisms, or at least all those who have a central nervous system have the same right to life and freedom from 'unnatural' exploitation and suffering (such a claim is highly contentious, since it presupposes that human actions are essentially 'unnatural'). To be more specific, it presupposes the possibility that humans and other sentient animals have the same moral status. If this is the case, then any use of animals for human purposes that involves suffering and/or death for the former would be immoral and ought thus to be avoided. The same goes for the closely related question, whether it is morally acceptable to alter the genome of animals to make xenotransplantation possible. This question presupposes the possibility that interfering with nature or with God's creations is bad, even if this involves no particular suffering.

In essence, there are two general ways of tackling these questions: either by appealing to philosophy, or by appealing to power (a combination of both may perhaps be seen as a third way, but it obviously gives primacy to power).

The classical philosophical argument that opposes abuse of animals for human needs, also called the 'antivivisectionist argument' insofar as it involves research on animals, proceeds from the assertion that there is no essential biological difference between some animals and humans. Whether true or false, this assertion purports to be a fact. In themselves, however, facts do not entail any moral implications or values. For example, the fact that 'Switzerland has a chocolate industry' does not in itself entail that 'Switzerland is good or bad', or indeed that 'chocolate is good or bad'. By the same token, the factual assumption that humans and other animals are biologically similar does not in itself entail any moral conclusion. In order to draw any moral conclusion, a general moral assertion needs to be added to the alleged fact. For example, if we asserted that 'countries that produce chocolate are good' or that 'sweets are good', then we could draw some moral conclusions based on our previous knowledge that 'Switzerland is a country' and that 'chocolate is a sweet'. Indeed, the antivivisectionist argument makes such a general moral assertion. It takes it for granted that 'the same should be treated the same' and deduces that humans ought not to do to animals things they would not want animals to do to them, if they could.[15]

The opposing argument may accept the claim about biological similarity, but it asserts that the moral status of humans is superior to that of all animals hence the former ought to exploit the latter if necessary. The argument is typically secular; however it may also draw on the Old Testament:

> And God said, Let us make man in our image, after our likeness: and let them have dominion over the fish of the sea, and over the fowl of the air, and over the cattle, and over all the earth, and over every creeping thing that creepeth upon the earth. So God created man in his own image, in the image of God created he him; male and female created he them. And God blessed them, and God said unto them, Be fruitful, and multiply, and replenish the earth, and subdue it: and have dominion over the fish of the sea, and over the fowl of the air, and over every living thing that moveth upon the earth (Genesis 1:26–28).

Like all philosophical debates, however, this one is also irresolvable. There cannot be any fundamental criterion that could tell us which of the opposing general moral premises is really true. This point is of great importance, for it actually entails that our choice to embrace one premise and reject the other was not made on the basis of any truth, but rather on the basis of our interests. The fact that, as a society, we do exploit animals reflects nothing but the dominance of those who have interests in the pertinent practices over those who have opposing interests.

This sociological conclusion sheds light on the second ethical question too: Ought animals to be protected from suffering while they are alive and when they are killed? Few would argue that we should not be concerned with the welfare of the animals. Some may argue that our moral duty to protect them from suffering is derived from their innate rights. Others may argue that such a duty is derived solely from concerns rather about the face and future of humanity. Whatever the case, the fact that it is now universally agreed that animals ought to be protected from suffering should not be seen as a victory of goodness over evil. Nor should it be seen as a reflection of the dominance of the antivivisectionists, let alone the animals themselves. On the contrary, it reflects a social compromise that rather reaffirms the domination of those who have some interest in exploiting animals. This conclusion may not make the philosophical debate redundant, but it strongly suggests that we should be more aware and perhaps even critical of the pertinent interests and the circumstances that have bred them.

2.3.2.3 *A financial bubble?*

So far, the paucity of practical achievements of research into xenotransplantation is in stark contrast to the amount of funding which the area attracts. In this respect, xenotransplantation resembles some other biomedical research areas, such as stem cell research and perhaps even the Human Genome Project as well. Nonmedical examples of practices that have had little value aside from increasing the GDP are well known, and are collectively called 'bubbles'. Of course, research into xenotransplantation may eventually prove to be fertile. However, its failure so far and the fact that it takes place when other alternatives are available should raise the questions whether it is not just another bubble and whether the money it absorbs should not be put to better use.

2.3.3 **Human organs**

At least as far as human organs are concerned, the history of transplant ethics is that of a continuous expansion. As mentioned above, the deepening organ crisis and the fact that the stakes are high for so many players explain why we have pushed, and continue to push, the ethical line to places that had previously been deemed immoral. Before we discuss the ethical debate around each of the historical-ethical milestones, it may be useful to observe the general trend first.

In the beginning we allowed deceased donations only. To tackle insufficient supply from the dead we embraced an increasingly inclusive definition of death. This has made it possible for us to retrieve organs from patients who had been considered legally alive according to the old definition of death. We then came up with the idea of opt-out consent according to which the dead are presumed to have given their consent for using their organs unless stated otherwise. These steps have certainly helped, but as the crisis continued to deepen we went one step further: we allowed donations from the living. In this category, we first permitted related and non-directed unrelated (anonymous) donations only. These measures have expanded the organ pool, but not enough.

By that time we had already become aware that interests in organ commerce were constantly intensifying, and that those in need of organs or money were increasingly likely to turn to the black market or seek a legal loophole that would allow them to conceal the commercial transaction behind some legitimate gesture. Until recently, we haven't done much about the black market, but we have banned altruistic-directed living unrelated donations of fear that they would become that legal loophole. This fear did not last long, though. The increasing hunger for more organs has driven us to legitimize this category as well. Indeed, it has helped a lot, but it did not suffice either. And so, still in the name of altruism and solidarity, we allowed paired exchange and donor chains. The contribution of these barter deals to the organ pool has only been marginal, though.

Recently, attempts to increase donation by removing disincentives (e.g. reimbursement of costs and assurance of free health care) or by offering noncommercial incentives (e.g. giving the relatives of a deceased donor priority on the transplant waiting list) are being considered in several countries. A thin line crosses between such measures and organ commercialism. Indeed, being tired of partial solutions, we are now introducing a dual strategy, depending on the audience: to those who still need to fool themselves we peddle the idea of quasi-noncommercial incentives for both living and deceased donations, and to those who no longer need to fool themselves we offer the bare market.

An educated assessment of trends and possibilities requires us to go back to the political economy of transplantation. That said, the prevailing trend is pretty obvious even without knowing much about it: if things are to continue as they have, we shall sooner or later embrace organ commercialism as one of the legitimate solutions to the underlying needs. The ethical justifications will follow the interests, not the other way around.

2.3.3.1 *Organs from the dead*

For some time, the dead used to be the almost exclusive source of organs for transplantation. This rested on three ethical premises. First, it is morally acceptable to retrieve organs, mainly kidneys, from the dead, if, when the subjects were still alive, they expressed their consent to donate their organs upon their death by signing a donor card or by making another form of advance directive. Second, it is morally acceptable to retrieve organs from the dead even without any advance directive, if their relatives gave their consent to donate their organs. Third, there is a fundamental moral difference between deceased and living donations: the former are morally acceptable, whereas the latter are not. There are two main reasons for this difference: the donation cannot harm the dead as much as it can harm the living, and the dead, unlike the living, are no longer at risk of donating their organs under coercion.

In an attempt to increase the organ pool without breaching the ethical premises of this category ethical amendments were made in relation to the definition of death (in most countries) in relation to the legal doctrine of consent (in some countries). The reader should again bear in mind that it was the underlying motivation that necessitated these ethical amendments, not the other way around. That said, whether or not they are philosophically plausible is for the reader to decide.

An expanding definition of death

Until the mid 1960s, death had been defined as the irreversible cessation of circulatory–respiratory function. The need to replace that definition with another became urgent when two economic interests appeared on the scene: interests in reducing the financial burden incurred by an increasing number of chronically ventilated comatose patients, and interests in retrieving organs for transplantation.[16] Regardless of any philosophical justification, this need was based on the understanding that expansion of the definition of death could legitimize withdrawal of ventilation and retrieval of organs, respectively, in some patients hitherto considered alive. In particular, an appropriate change in the definition of death could, if embraced by the law, legitimize retrieval of hearts from patients who, according to the then prevailing definition had been considered alive, that is to say, brain-dead patients whose circulatory functions are maintained even if by mechanical means only.

The concept of 'brain death' was canonized soon after the publication of the report of the Harvard Committee in 1968.[17] In the opening remarks, the committee, on which two transplant surgeons sat, was very clear about the interests underlying its endorsement of the concept — meeting the increasing demand for organs, and containing the financial crisis in intensive care and dialysis. These interests were later reiterated even more explicitly by the founder of the committee himself, the famous doctor, Henry Beecher.[18] Interestingly, the report made no reference to any neurological research and was totally unclear about the very criteria of brain death. Moreover, it did not take the trouble to conceal the role of the new definition and its underlying interests behind any philosophical justification. This was first done by the President's Commission in 1981, only following a heated public controversy.[19] The philosophical rationale underlying the new definition was simple: human life requires cognition; cognition, hence human life, resides in a functioning brain; hence brain death and only brain death means death.

Though the change in the definition of death initially increased the organ pool, its practical implications were limited. Firstly, pronouncement of death based on brain death criteria could apply in certain hospital settings only. Secondly, the required neurological tests have proved to be expensive. Thus in order to overcome these limitations, an even more flexible definition of death was called upon: when pronouncing death, doctors are now encouraged to *choose* between brain death and circulatory-respiratory death, depending on the circumstances, and the interests. Accordingly, the death of hospital patients who are not potential donors is established by the criteria of the old definition, and the same goes for non-hospital patients who are potential donors.

In 2007, the *Washington Post* reported that doctors were increasingly declaring patients dead within minutes after their heart stopped beating and without any evidence of brain death, so that surgeons could remove their organs.[20] This trend is openly supported by major figures in the American transplant community, notwithstanding claims that the presumption that the act of organ procurement has taken place after death (the 'dead donor rule') is a legal fiction.[21,22]

The concept of 'legal fiction' invites a brief explication, since, as we shall see, it plays a central role in several practices in transplantation where it raises some serious ethical questions.

With minor differences in formulation, most modern law dictionaries define legal fiction as a presumption taken to be true by the courts of law, irrespective of whether it is true or false, and even though it might knowingly be false. Not every presumption is a legal fiction, though. To be a legal fiction, the chances that a presumption be true must be significantly diminished. In principle, this may happen when the presumption does not lend itself to scrutiny, let alone serious scrutiny, and where circumstantial conditions that make it somewhat unlikely to be true apply.[23]

In view of the underlying interests and the difficulty in establishing the facts, the presumption that 'death has occurred prior to the retrieval of the organs' may indeed be a legal fiction. In strong words, it may become a legal loophole that conceals murder. Precisely for the same reasons, the presumption that 'the pronouncement of death is done independently of the retrieval of the organs' also turns out to be legal fiction.

We may believe that there is nothing wrong with retrieving organs from cadavers. But in view of what's been said, wouldn't we feel more comfortable if we knew that our current definitions and criteria of death remained in place even under a political economy that contained no economic interests in death?[24]

Opt-out consent

The legal doctrine of informed consent provides the justification for retrieving organs from those who have the mental capacity to consent as long as they are informed and can make a free and voluntary choice. As long as these conditions apply, the doctrine is not concerned about whether the consent was explicit (opt-in consent) or implicit/presumed (opt-out consent).

In most cases, consent to donate one's organs when one dies or consent to donate the organs of a deceased relative is of the opt-in kind. The subjects involved must give their explicit consent to donate the organs. In other words, their organs will not be taken without such consent. However, several countries have introduced and others are considering introducing a system of opt-out consent. In such a system, people are presumed to have given their consent to become organ donors after death, unless they explicitly refused.

The effect of an opt-out system on deceased donation rates is difficult to establish, since so many other factors are also involved. Such factors include the nonexistence or existence of efficient donor programmes, the level of public trust in the medical authorities and its motivations, and general cultural attitudes toward deceased donation. Indeed, in Spain and Greece, two countries that have an opt-out system in action, the trends are opposite: the donation rates in Spain are high while those in Greece are low. In fact, there is some evidence that under certain social conditions the opt-out system can have a detrimental effect of donation rates. The UK, for example, has recently rejected proposals to introduce such a system precisely because of such fears.[25]

These are mainly empirical concerns, not ethical ones. The ethical rationale behind the opt-out system draws on the presumption that all people are willing to donate their organs after death, but some are simply too lazy to give their explicit consent. This presumption can be put in other words: those who did not sign a donor card, would have signed it, had they been less lazy. The aim of an opt-out system is thus to bypass the laziness of individuals, not their free will.

Interestingly, the idea of opt-out consent has only rarely attracted criticism for being immoral. This is notwithstanding the fact that the presumption upon which it is based is just another instance of legal fiction. Opt-out consent does not necessarily imply consent, let alone informed consent. It may increase the organ pool by recruiting many who are really willing to donate their organs, but it might also recruit those who are not. In part, then, this system is effectively based on deception.

State ownership of deceased organs

A far more extreme version of the opt-out system is the idea that deceased organs should be owned by the state and made use of regardless of the wishes of the subjects involved.[26] Like the opt-out system, such a proposal could be justified only if it rested upon a total social consensus. Such a consensus does not exist as of yet.

Deceased organ commercialism

Currently, commerce in deceased organs is illegal in all countries, and is thus confined to the black market. Nevertheless, proposals to legalize the practice have been made in an attempt to exhaust the procurement potential of this category. These proposals offer some material value to families who are willing to vend (the term 'donate' is inappropriate in this case) their deceased relative's organs. This material value could be translated, for example, to life insurance, covering funeral costs, obtaining priority in the transplant waiting list for needy family members, and even cash payments.

Deceased organ commercialism poses some serious ethical issues. How-ever, these shall be discussed in the next section that deals with, among others, living organ commercialism. The latter, so it will be argued, raises precisely the same issues.[27,28]

2.3.3.2 *Organs from the living*

The benefits of using organs from the living, mainly kidney and liver, over deceased organs are prominent. This organ pool is potentially bigger; the transplantation may be planned in advance; the quality of the organ and its suitability for the particular recipient, hence the survival of the graft, are generally better. This general category raises two major ethical issues, however.

First, one should note that procurement of organs from the living is an act of medicalization, namely, an act that imposes the categories and practices of medicine on a nonmedical object. Indeed, this act requires us to abandon the supreme Hippocratic principle according to which it is essentially unprofessional to turn a healthy person, i.e. the donor, into a patient, even if for a short time only. To justify this audacious step we appeal to the deontological principle of respect for the donor's autonomy and the legal doctrine of informed consent, and to the utilitarian premise of maximization of happiness (both the donor and the recipient are happier than before). Unfortunately, however, there is no fundamental philosophical criterion that could tell us which of the two ethics is 'really' moral and which is 'really' immoral (theoretically, both may be immoral, but if one is moral, then the other must be immoral). One thing should be clear, though: we have made the ethical choice on the basis of our historically evolving interests.

And yet a difficult ethical question should be raised in this context: if indeed it is morally acceptable for a doctor to take out the kidney of a healthy person based on a certain ethic, should it not be also morally acceptable to take out his or her heart based on the same ethic?

We currently say no. We believe that there is an essential difference between the cases as the latter inevitably entails death. We still feel that doctors ought not to deliberately kill people under any circumstances. On the other hand, there are signs that the idea of physician–assisted suicide is gaining popularity in many societies, and that in such cases the ethical justification appeals to the principle of respect for the patient's autonomy. Why then should a mother who wants to donate her heart to her son be treated differently?

The answer cannot be found in ethics, but in sociology. The political economy of assisted suicide is different from that of living heart donation. One day, if our interests dictate so, the stubborn remnant of the Hippocratic ethics, which still affects the latter category, may disappear.

The general category of living donation raises another ethical issue: the demand for organs may put healthy people at risk of losing their organs under some form of coercion. Organ robbery is an extreme example. However, coerced 'donation' can also occur in the presence of the donor's informed consent. In other words, informed consent in itself does not rule out coercion. This unfortunate fact has been widely recognized, and attempts have indeed been made to ban practices that involve coercion even regardless of the presence of consent. Whether these attempts were effective or not is a completely different matter, however.

Related donation and non-directed unrelated (anonymous) donation

In order to prevent forms of coercion that might be concealed behind informed consent, we first allowed related donation and non-directed unrelated (anonymous) donation only. We have assumed that family ties and non-directedness preclude coercion and necessarily imply altruism. This assumption is another form of a legal fiction, however. In fact, the mechanisms that we installed to confirm that assumption are lax. They do not allow certain forms of coercion to interfere with the donor's consent. For example, the subtle forms of coercion that might occur within the family are often overlooked by the prevailing control mechanisms. The tendency of wives and husbands to become donors and recipients, respectively, which has been mentioned above, reflects this failure fairly well. A similar problem exists in the case of non-directed unrelated donations. Such donations seem to preclude coercion even better than related donations, but even they cannot preclude complex clandestine commercial ties, which as we shall see, presuppose and imply some sort of coercion. In this case too, the prevailing control mechanisms are usually unable to spot any commercial ties.

Altruistic-directed unrelated donations

This subcategory of living donation has been banned for a long time of fear that the presumption of altruism could become a legal loophole concealing clandestine commercial ties between vendor and emptor, hence some form of coercion. This fear is not baseless. The deepening organ crisis, the decline of social solidarity, and the evolving interests in organ commercialism are likely to turn this presumption into a legal fiction.

Nevertheless, the increasing demand for organs has made us abandon that fear. In most countries this subcategory is now acceptable.[29] Control mechanisms have indeed been installed, but they too are somewhat lax. For example, the control mechanisms in the United States and in Israel are fairly similar in rigour.[30] However, comparisons of the socioeconomic profile of donors versus recipients in both countries suggest that these mechanisms are more likely to be fooled in Israel. This strongly suggests that the factors that determine whether altruistic-directed unrelated donation becomes a legal fiction or not should not be sought in the rigour of the control mechanism, but rather in the strength of the local social solidarity.[31]

Paired exchange and donor chains

Related donations may not always be the best option even if potential coercion is not an issue. Indeed, donor-recipient incompatibility will rule out such donation. Recently, creative solutions were developed to bypass this problem. For example, if fathers X and Y want to donate their kidneys to their sons x and y, respectively, but their kidneys could only be given to y and x, respectively, then a paired exchange may take place. X will give his kidney to y, and Y will give his one to x. Similarly, an extended chain may be formed, involving more than two donors. Moreover, a donor chain may involve not just donors and their related recipients, but also altruistic donors who have no designated recipients and thus do not expect to receive anything in return.[32]

Such enterprises obviously require meticulous technical logistics. However, they are also required to prevent breach of the group contract by one or more of the candidate donors. In the case of a paired exchange, such a breach could be prevented by having all four operations done simultaneously. Since simultaneity is almost impossible in the case of a long donor chain (the completion of the chain could sometimes take several months), the ethical challenge is more difficult and could be partly overcome by the recruitment of altruistic donors who have no designated recipients.

This subcategory of living donations has been hailed as a perfectly ethical solution, not just because it is based on the consent of the participants, but also because it increases social solidarity. Paradoxically, however, proponents of organ commercialism may argue that it serves as a pretext for the idea they wish to push through. Based on the claims that (1) paired exchange and donor chains are private instances of barter, that (2) barter is ethically acceptable, and that (3) money simply facilitates barter by giving the players more freedom, they could argue that all transactions that involve money, buying and selling of organs included, ought to be ethically acceptable too. Moreover, they could add that the risk of trading one's kidney for too little money is no greater than the risk involved in trading one's good kidney for one of lesser quality.

The analogy between barter in organs and commerce in organs may fall flat, however. In the former case one kidney is traded for another kidney, while in the latter case the kidney is traded for another commodity. This difference in itself does not have a moral significance, but the difference in the circumstances underlying each of these transactions may indeed have a moral significance.

Organ commercialism

As we have seen, the political economy of the organ crisis breeds pressures to commercialize organ procurement. As a matter of fact, in the current situation each and every stakeholder has some interest in a market in organs. Both those who need the organs as well as those who need the money can expect the market to be able to meet their respective needs. At the same time, some of the stakeholders have opposing interests as well. For example, potential vendors who have an interest in trading their kidney for money also have an interest in not having to make such a choice in the first place. The same goes for patients who have an interest in buying a kidney. It is not a great pleasure to have to sell or buy body parts.

This conflict of interests is reflected in the global legal reality. On the one hand, almost all countries still forbid commerce in organs (Iran is currently the only exception) with a black market existing in some parts of the world. On the other hand, the voices that call for legalization of some form of organ commercialism intensify. Interestingly, however, both the opponents and the proponents of organ commercialism are unified on one point: transplant tourism, where a patient from a rich country travels to buy a kidney in a poor country, and other forms of the black market are not just immoral but also deleterious as far as local interests are concerned. This position has been asserted by several international bodies.[33–35]

The current debate around organ commercialism takes place between those who oppose any form of organ commercialism and those who support some form of local commercialism. This debate reflects a conflict of interests within the political economy of transplantation, but it takes place in the realm of ethics.

1. The pro-market argument

The pro-market discourse maintains that, however efficient, a transplant donor programme that appeals to social solidarity and the goodwill of individuals will inevitably fail to meet the increasing demand for organs. It asserts that letting patients suffer and die on the waiting lists, when so many organs are out there just begging to be harvested, is morally unacceptable, and so is wasting public resources. Noncommercial systems are thus both ineffective as well as immoral.

The pro-market discourse holds that, in contrast, the market, and only the market, can provide unlimited access to these organs and be moral at the same time. Not any market, though. A global organ market, for example, is not just counterproductive but also immoral. This is because it creates severe inequities in the distribution of power, benefit and risk. Such faults, the discourse contends, result from the essentially unfettered nature of this market. A global organ market cannot be tamed and is thus bound to remain both counterproductive as well as immoral.

That said, an organ market that is free from any practical drawbacks and inequities is feasible within the bounds of a national market or an economic union. It must adhere to certain regulatory principles, though. As far as the protection of recipients is concerned, such principles include a single buyer, mechanisms assuring safety and quality, and systems that guarantee equitable, non-means-based allocation of the organs. The principles are no less attentive to the welfare of the vendors. In addition to the single buyer, they include mechanisms validating consent requirements, safeguards against buying organs from vulnerable people, strict prohibition of brokering, and systems assuring competitive remuneration, life insurance, continuous health care, and priority in transplant waiting lists.[36]

Otherwise, the pro-market discourse sees no essential moral problem with trading in organs. Firstly, body parts are private property. In the name of liberty, their owners should be free to do with them as they like. Secondly, both parties can make a free choice, at least in principle. The unpleasant nature of the dilemma each one of them is facing does not by itself make their choices unfree. On the contrary, it is rather the existing prohibition of commerce in organs that limits their freedom, often with dire consequences for both of them. Thirdly, the generally accurate classification of buyers and vendors as rich and poor, respectively, may perhaps seem to reflect inequities and suggest relations of power and exploitation. However, this does not have to be the case. In the regulated market, the parties would maintain perfectly symmetrical relations vis-à-vis each other. Their complementary deficiencies and surpluses would guarantee 'mutual exploitation' and hence equal distribution of benefits and risks. Fourthly, many instances involving commerce in the body are already legitimate. Making the kidney an exception would be ethically inconsistent. Fifthly, the real choice we are facing, and the only one, is between a regulated market and a black market. Considering the interests of buyers and vendors, the former is by far the better option.

2. The anti-market argument

The argument against a regulated market in organs makes two points. First, it casts doubt upon its feasibility and efficacy. It maintains that regulation would be counterproductive, if not altogether impossible. With so much money at stake, it posits, the regulatory mechanisms that purport to assure liberty, quality and safety are bound to fail, doctor–patient relationships would be harmed, and people would start buying what they currently get for free, which would increase public spending.

Being empirical in nature, these claims have a clear advantage over ethical ones: they appeal to reason, not sentiment. They may even attempt to appeal to the reason of the proponents of the market themselves. Otherwise, they are disturbing. Firstly, the political economy of transplantation indicates that some players have vested interests in the organ market regardless of whether it is regulated or not. These powerful players do not care about any other consequences. They are unlikely to be convinced. Secondly, such claims presuppose that there is actually nothing wrong with the ideally regulated market, hence with the fundamental principle of trade in body parts. As such, they effectively normalize and moralize the commercial idea. Finally, to argue that the regulated market is bound to fail when one believes that the experiment carries a high risk is a very dangerous thing to do. Indeed, empirical claims do not scare the proponents of the market. In fact, they invite them to try to prove their case, and they will not turn this invitation down.

To be robust, then, the anti-market discourse should not be concerned with the feasibility or the efficacy of a regulated market. On the contrary, it should take its premises at face value, and direct its criticism at the very heart of the problem — principle of trade in body parts.

Indeed, the second point which the argument makes addresses the bare principle of trade in body parts. In attempt to identify its moral fault, it points at the payment as the source of evil. Indeed, it associates a greater payment with greater coercion and a smaller payment with greater exploitation. It uses this culprit to conclude that since the payment violates the human dignity of the vendor, a ban thereon would preserve that dignity.

However, this is fundamentally wrong. In the ideally-regulated organ market there is a complementary symmetry between emptor and vendor. Every buyer is also a seller, and every seller is also a buyer. One buys a kidney and sells money, while the other buys money and sells a kidney. Moreover, each of the commodities in question is the equivalent of the other. Under such circumstances it would be unreasonable to describe any one of the offers as being coercive, let alone more coercive than the other. Indeed, no one would describe an offer to sell one's kidney in terms of 'undue inducement', so why should one describe an offer to sell one's money in such terms?

If this is still not convincing, one could make a different argument, such that is not based on assumptions about any symmetry, equivalence, or any exchange. Imagine a worker in a meat factory whose hand has just got stuck in a giant mincer that threatens to devour him completely. The switch is located in another room, so that the machine could not be deactivated quickly enough to save the poor man's life. The only thing one could do is offer him the nearest knife so that he could choose whether he wants to cut himself free from his hand or not.

Now, would you describe this offer as coercive? Would you argue that the sharper the knife the more coercive the offer, or that the blunter it is the more exploitative the offer? Would your answers to these questions depend on the interests or motivations of the helper? Certainly not! What you could do is acknowledge that the offer gives the worker a choice, and that giving him that choice, however sad, is better than giving him no choice at all.

We shall return to this gruesome scenario in a moment, but let us first see that neither organ commerce nor an embargo thereon has anything to do with the human dignity of the vendor.

Anatole France (1844–1924), the French poet and novelist and the Nobel laureate for literature for 1921, wrote: 'The law, in its majestic equality, forbids the rich as well as the poor to sleep under bridges, to beg in the streets, and to steal bread.'[37] Now let us portray a different law, such that allows both the rich and the poor to sleep under bridges etc. According to the anti-market conclusion the former law respects the human dignity of the subjects in question, whereas the latter does not. The truth is that none of these laws is better than the other. If there is any problem with the respective social systems, then it resides in the difference between rich and poor as far as their available options are concerned, and in the fact that none of these laws addresses that difference.

But if payment for organs is not in itself morally problematic, what then is wrong with trade in body parts?

To answer this question, let us go back to our meat-factory scenario and look deeper into the context. We might perhaps discover that the calamity was neither the worker's own fault nor was it the result of any natural or supernatural decree. As a matter of fact, our worker, whether he be the rich patient who needs a kidney or the poor person who has nothing to sell but his kidney, was deliberately pushed into the mincer. Indeed, the political economy of our society shows that both kidney failure as well as poverty are largely the outcomes of certain social practices which are propelled by certain beneficiaries. Now, if this is where the evil exists, then the offer of the knife, and in our case the offer of money for a kidney and vice versa, will no longer seem to be morality incarnate. It will transpire to be just an ethical façade that conceals and reaffirms an underlying immorality.

To be robust, then, the anti-market argument should acknowledge the fact that the regulated market is ethical and reject it precisely on that ground.

It should tell its audience that those who push some people into kidney disease and others into poverty ought not to be allowed to hide these wrongs behind any ethical veil. To those who are rightly concerned with the fate of the individual person who begs for an acute solution to it should explain that the suffering-preventing capacity of a kidney disease-free and poverty-free world is considerably greater than that of any organ market.

To conclude this part of the chapter let us focus again on the difference between organ donation and organ vending. In the former case, the donor cares very much about the fate of the organ once it has been removed from his or her body. In the latter case, the vendor becomes *alienated* to the organ. He or she no longer cares about its fate; on the contrary, many vendors actually wish that it be rejected! Such alienation reflects heteronomy (the opposite of autonomy), hence some form of coercion.

This point has bearing on both living and deceased organ commercialism: in both cases, the vendors would not have sold the organs had they not been deprived of better options. Neither the problem nor its solution should be sought in the market ethics, but rather in the social factors that inflict this deprivation and thereby drive the victims to seek refuge in the market.[38]

2.4 The Ethical Discourse: Distribution of Organs

2.4.1 Prosthetic implants

The distribution of prosthetic implants raises several general and specific ethical issues. Social equity is a general issue. It does not depend on the specific nature of the implant/organ but rather on whether its distribution is regulated by the free market or by the public health care system. With small differences in emphasis, a similar issue exists in the distribution of organs obtained from animal and human sources as well.

Distribution of implants and organs, which is regulated by market forces only, that is to say, by the purchasing capacity of the patients, would mean that only the relatively rich could have access to the treatment. This begs the general question whether such treatments ought to be treated like any other commodity or be given to the needy regardless of their financial status. The answer to this question requires a profound analysis of the prevailing political economy of production in general. This goes beyond the scope of this paper, but two central points can be made. If the analysis were to show that all goods, including implants, have been produced by society, one could argue that they should also be owned and distributed by society and not by private individuals who, because of class relations of power, happen to appropriate them. Equally, if the analysis were to show that the class of private owners of commodities were also responsible for the emergence of production- and consumption-related diseases, then it should take responsibility at least for treating the victims. If medical treatment is a human right, then this is only because of that reason.

But the distribution of implants and organs may raise an ethical problem even when regulated by the public. If implants and organs are scarce, how should we allocate them? The basic approach has been based on the principle of 'first come, first served' (ignoring the need) and need (ignoring the place in the waiting list). Recently, however, criteria of outcome were also introduced. In some cases, these are replacing the criterion of need. For example, hip replacement, which requires an implant, is often allocated to those who are likely to show better outcomes, namely, those who are not obese. It is denied from those who need it most. This utilitarian value-for-money approach seems to be compatible with a good investment policy, but it is ethically dubious. It discriminates against the obese, whose condition is now known to result from certain forms of social consumption. The system that has made these people ill exempts itself from responsibility for their care.

A different question that may emerge in the case of implants is if and when the device should be turned off. This question, which applies particularly to life-sustaining implants, belongs to the realm of end-of-life ethics.

Another ethical issue concerns the potential capacity of electronic implants to replace lost neurological functions or enhance human capabilities beyond normal levels. In the case of replacement of lost functions — cochlear and ocular implants, for example — problems of adaptation may exist. As far as the case of enhanced capabilities is concerned, this capacity is still largely fictional. However, mental changes and changes in personal identity have been named as potential risks. One may also argue that there should be a limit to any enhancement, but the real question is that of benefit and loss, beneficiaries and victims.

2.4.2 **Xenogeneic organs**

In the case of xenotransplantation, the issue of social equity receives a specific dimension, because the service might become available only within the confines of private health care, and yet it might expose the entire population to the risk of infection by known and unknown agents. This injustice is still more disturbing to the extent that public resources are being mobilized to develop xenotransplantation.

There may also be some cultural barriers, primarily religious, to receiving xenogeneic organs. However, these may be overcome by other alternatives, and possibly by reinterpretation of the underlying taboos.

2.4.3 **Human organs**

The problem of social equity is of primary concern in this area. In non-commercial settings, a combination of waiting list, need, outcome, tissue compatibility and the quality of the available organs forms the acceptable way of allocating the organs. Even the idea of a regulated market in organs accepts this premise (in contrast, a 'free' market in organs allocates them only according to the purchasing capacity of the customer). 'Need' and 'outcome' are very delicate issues, however. Are the young in greater need than the elderly? Should those whose prognosis is worse be discriminated against?

Let us consider one case only. Two patients are waiting for a liver transplant, but only one liver is available. One has an idiopathic liver disease, and the other has alcoholic liver cirrhosis. Everything else is equal. We know that the prognosis of the latter patient is worse, let alone that he or she are likely to resume drinking. Who should receive the liver?

Currently, our common intuition would give the priority to the patient whose lifestyle has played no role in the pathophysiology of the underlying condition. This is not surprising, since we tend to think in categories of 'outcome' and 'personal responsibility'. Alcoholism, however, is a social problem. In part it has cultural features, but in part it is also caused by profit-driven and perhaps even politically driven forms of consumption. If this is the case, then the latter patient should be seen as a victim of society. Denying the transplant from this patient would thus double the injustice.

A closely related issue concerns the effect of the time spent on the waiting list on the outcomes of transplantation. We know that the longer the wait, the poorer the prognosis. Criteria of outcome would therefore prioritize those who have entered the list just recently. In turn, those who have been waiting a long time would have to wait even longer.

Transplantation of organs from human sources raises two other issues of justice and fairness. The first issue concerns the suggestion that patients should receive a transplant only if they have been willing to donate their own organs upon their death. This idea is found seriously wanting, since it has the potential of discriminating against those who are unaware of donor programmes, and those who have some cultural or political (distrust in medical authorities) reason for not signing a donor card. Under such circumstances, the idea of conditionality becomes just another form of social victimization.

An extension of the idea of conditionality can be found in suggestions to give priority to relatives of a deceased donor. Such suggestions, which are usually marketed as noncommercial incentives for donation, have the capacity of discriminating against patients on the waiting list who have had no deceased donor in their family.

Another issue to be mentioned here concerns allocation of organs to foreigners. In the context of transplant tourism, such allocation is known to have a detrimental effect on noncommercial patients in both countries involved. In the context of some international agreement it is acceptable, however. For example, two or more countries may have an organ-sharing programme on the basis of equality. Equally, one country that has a developed transplant system may help another country that has no such system.

However, by far the biggest and the most disturbing problem concerns the global inequity in access to transplantation. We typically mention the numbers on the transplant waiting lists in developed countries. However, we tend to forget that most patients who suffer from organ failure can only dream of dialysis, let alone a waiting list. The solution to this problem will not be found in the globalization of commerce, but rather in the globalization of wealth and freedom.

References

1. Organ Procurement and Transplantation Network. (2009). Available at: http://optn.transplant.hrsa.gov/ (accessed 9 August 2010).
2. NHS Blood and Transplant. (2011). *Transplant Activity in the UK 2010–2011*. Available at: http://www.uktransplant.org.uk/ukt/statistics/transplant_activity_report/transplant_activity_report.jsp (accessed 27 July 2011).
3. About Operations. (2011). *Organ Donation: Facts and Figures*. Available at: http://www.aboutoperations.co.uk/organ-donation-facts-figures.html (accessed 1 September 2010).
4. Sagmeister, M. *et al.* (2002). Cost-Effectiveness of Cadaveric and Living-donor Liver Transplantation, *Transplantation*, **73(4)**, 616–622.
5. NHS Blood and Transplant. (2009). *Cost-effectiveness of Transplantation*. Available at: http://www.uktransplant.org.uk/ukt/newsroom/fact_sheets/cost_effectiveness_of_transplantation.jsp (accessed 13 March 2011).
6. Gal, I. (2009). Heart Recipient's Father: We'll Never Donate Organs, *Israel Jewish Scene*. Available at: http://www.ynet.co.il/english/articles/0,7340,1-3663653,00.html (accessed 12 May 2010).
7. Scheper-Hughes, N. (2007). The Tyranny of the Gift: Sacrificial Violence in Living Donor Transplants, *Am J Transplant*, **7(3)**, 507–511.
8. Budiani-Saberi, D.A. and Delmonico, F.L. (2008). Response to: Will Transplant Tourism Erode the Surgical Skills of Transplant Surgeons in Israel? *Am J Transplant*, **8**, 1964.
9. Israel Transplant Law. (2008). [17/68, in Hebrew.] Available at: http://www.knesset.gov.il/privatelaw/data/17/3/68_3_1.tf (accessed 1 March 2011).
10. Hobbes, T. (1996 [1651]). *Leviathan*, Oxford University Press, Oxford, I.11.21.
11. Gramsci, A. (1971). *Selection from the Prison Notebooks*, Lawrence & Wishart, London.
12. Hansson, S.O. (2005). Implant Ethics, *J Med Ethics*, **31**, 519–525.
13. Marcuse, H. (2002 [1964]). *One-Dimensional Man: Studies in the Ideology of Advanced Industrial Society*, Routledge, London.
14. Collignon, P. and Purdy, L. (2001). Xenografts: Are the Risks so Great that We Should Not Proceed? *Microbes Infect*, **3**, 341–348.
15. Singer, P. (2009). *Animal Liberation: The Definitive Classic of the Animal Movement*, Harper Perennial, New York.
16. Wolstenholme, G. and O'Connor, M. (eds.) (1966). *Ciba Foundation Symposium. Ethics in Medical Progress*, J & A Churchill Ltd, London.
17. No author. (1968). Report of the Ad Hoc Committee of the Harvard Medical School to Examine the Definition of Brain Death: A Definition of Irreversible Coma, *JAMA*, **205**, 337–340.
18. Beecher, H. (1969). Scarce Resources and Medical Advancement: Ethical Aspects of Experimentation with Human Subjects, *Daedalus*, **98(2)**, 275–313.

19. President's Commission on Ethical Problems in Medicine and Biomedical and Behavioral Research. (1981). *Defining Death: A Report on Medical, Legal, and Ethical Issues in the Definition of Death*, U.S. Government Printing Office, Washington, D.C.

20. Stein, R. (2007). New Trend in Organ Donation Raises Questions, *Washington Post*, 18 March, A03. Available at: http://www.washingtonpost.com/wp-dyn/content/article/2007/03/17/AR2007031700963.html (accessed 10 February 2011).

21. Rady, M.Y., Verheijde, J.L. and McGregor, J. (2006). Organ Donation After Cardiocirculatory Death and the Dead Donor Rule: What is the Evidence? *Can Med Assoc J eLetters*, 30 October. Available at: http://www.cmaj.ca/content/175/8/S1/reply#cmaj_el_5442?sid=0ae6bf94-fd24-4f28-b90d-508d701126fe (accessed 25 January 2011).

22. Steinbrook, R. (2007). Organ Donation after Cardiac Death, *NEJM*, **357(3)**, 209–213.

23. Epstein, M. (2007). Legal and Institutional Fictions in Medical Ethics: A Common, and Yet Largely Overlooked, Phenomenon, *J Med Ethics*, **33(6)**, 362–364.

24. Epstein, M. (2009). The Political Economy of Death and the History of Its Criteria, *Rev Neurosci*, **20(3–4)**, 293–297.

25. Department of Health. (2008). The Potential Impact of an Opt-Out System for Organ Donation in the UK: An Independent Report from the Organ Donation Taskforce. Available at: http://www.dh.gov.uk/en/Publicationsandstatistics/Publications/PublicationsPolicyAndGuidance/DH_090312 (accessed 3 May 2011).

26. Schönfeld, M.R. (1994–1995). Whose Tissues Are They Anyway? A Proposal for State Ownership of the Human Body and Its Parts, *J Cardiovasc Diagn Proced*, **12(3)**, 145–149.

27. Mayrhofer-Reinhartshuber, D. and Fitzgerald, R. (2004). Financial Incentives for Cadaveric Organ Donation, *Ann Transplant*, **9(1)**, 25–27.

28. Arnold, R. *et al.* (2002). Financial Incentives for Cadaver Organ Donation: An Ethical Reappraisal, *Transplantation*, **73**, 1361–1367.

29. Directive 2004/23/EC of the European Parliament and of the Council of 31 March 2004 on Setting Standards of Quality and Safety for the Donation, Procurement, Testing, Processing, Preservation, Storage and Distribution of Human Tissues and Cells.

30. Dew, M.A. *et al.* (2007). Guidelines for the Psychosocial Evaluation of Living Unrelated Kidney Donors in the United States, *Am J Transplant*, **7**, 1047–1054.

31. Epstein, M. and Danovitch, G.M. (2009). Is Altruistic Directed Living Unrelated Organ Donation a Legal Fiction? *Nephrol Dial Transpl*, **24**, 357–360.

32. Rees, M.A. *et al.* (2009). A Nonsimultaneous, Extended, Altruistic-Donor Chain, *NEJM*, **360(11)**, 1096–1101.

33. World Health Organization. (2008). *WHO Guiding Principles on Human Cell, Tissue and Organ Transplantation*, EB 123/5, May 26.

34. Steering Committee of the Istanbul Summit. (2008). Organ Trafficking and Transplant Tourism and Commercialism: The Declaration of Istanbul, *Lancet*, **372**, 5–6.

35. Epstein, M. (2009). Sociological and Ethical Issues in Transplant Commercialism, *Curr Opin Organ Tran*, **14(2)**, 134–139.

36. Erin, C.A. and Harris, J. (1994). 'A Monopsonistic Market: Or How to Buy and Sell Human Organs, Tissues and Cells Ethically', in Robinson, I. (ed.), *Life and Death Under High-Technology Medicine*, Manchester University Press in association with the Fulbright Commission, London, pp. 134–153.

37. France, A. (1930 [1894]). *The Red Lily*, The Bodley Head, London, Chapter 7.

38. Epstein, M. (2007). The Ethics of Poverty and the Poverty of Ethics: The Case of Palestinian Prisoners in Israel Seeking to Sell their Kidneys in Order to Feed Their Children, *J Med Ethics*, **33**, 473–474.

3

HLA, The Human Major Histocompatibility Complex

Jacques Colombani

The name "major histocompatibility complex" (MHC) indicates the capacity of its products to induce a strong allogeneic immune response, particularly in the context of transplantation. This property was at the origin of the discovery of the MHC in the mouse (histocompatibility-2; H-2) and in man (human leukocyte antigen: HLA), a property which permitted its study using immunogenetic methods. However, the natural biological function of the MHC is to present antigen fragments (peptides) to T lymphocytes. The MHC can therefore be defined as a group of molecules involved in the presentation of peptides to the T cell receptor (TCR). This definition concerns antigen–presenting molecules and also other molecules which may contribute to the presentation function. This functional definition is completed by a genetic definition of the MHC as the chromosome region which contains the genes controlling the structure and expression of antigen–presenting molecules (Figure 3.1). The two definitions are complementary, but somewhat different. It is indeed possible for MHC products to exercise functions other than presentation. Further, it is clear that many genes located in the MHC are only fortuitously associated, without any relationship with the presentation function. Others, such as TAP (transporter of antigen peptides), TNF (tumor necrosis factor) or HSP (heat shock protein)

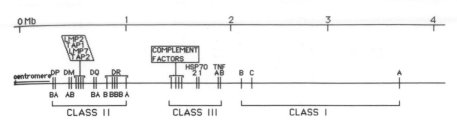

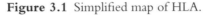

Figure 3.1 Simplified map of HLA.

The HLA complex is located on the short arm of chromosome 6 (6p21.3). It extends over about 3.5 Mb. Class I and class II genes code the protein chains of corresponding molecules. Three MHC1 molecules, HLA-A, B, C, are expressed at the membrane of most nucleated cells in the organism. Many other class I and class-like genes (20–30) have been identified. Most of these are pseudogenes; some may be expressed in small quantities and/or only in certain tissues. Class II genes encode the α(HLA-DRA, DQA1, DPA1) and β chains (HLA-DRB1, B3, B4, B5, DQB1, DPB1) of class II molecules. Three or four molecules are encoded by an HLA haplotype: one DP molecule (DPA1 and DPB1 genes), one DQ molecule (DQA1 and DQB1 genes) and one or two DR molecules. One DR molecule (DRA and DRB1 genes) is always expressed. A second DR molecule (DRA gene and DRB3, B4 or B5 gene) is usually expressed. In certain HLA haplotypes, there is no second functional DRB gene and therefore no second molecule expressed. DMA and DMB genes code for a DM molecule expressed in an intracytoplasmic compartment, where it contributes to peptide loading on classical MHC2 molecules. DOA and DOB genes code for a DO molecule which modulates the peptide loading activity of HLA-DM in the endocytic pathway.[1]

Numerous other genes are associated to genes coding membrane HLA molecules. Class III genes encode three (C2, Bf, C4) of the 20 or so complement factors in this non-specific immune defence system. HSP70-1 and 2 encode two proteins (heat shock protein) which protect cell proteins during stress. They may play the role of chaperone proteins during the assembly of MHC1 and 2 molecules. TNFA encodes the TNFα (cachectin), a cytokine produced by monocytes and macrophages. Endowed with lytic activity, it increases the expression of class I and II HLA genes. TNFB encodes the TNFβ (lymphotoxin), a cytokine close to but distinct from TNFα, and produced by T lymphocytes.

TAP1 and 2 encode two homologous proteins which associate to form a heterodimer (TAP: transporter of antigen peptides), functioning as a peptide pump inserted in the membrane of the endoplasmic reticulum. LMP2 and 7 code two of the 16–20 proteins making up the proteasome (LMP: large multifunctional protease), a proteolytic structure present in the cytosol (Figure 3.4). Tapasin gene code for a 48 kDa chaperone protein playing an important role in the formation of the peptide loading complex which loads peptide on MHC1.[2]

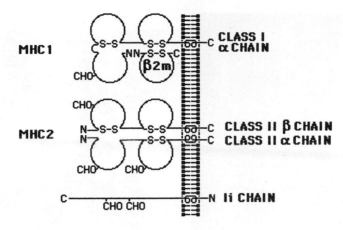

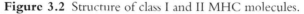

Figure 3.2 Structure of class I and II MHC molecules.

The class I molecule is a transmembrane glycoprotein comprising a heavy chain α(44 kDa), bound non-covalently with a non-glycosylated light chain (11.5 kDa), β2 microglobulin (β2m), which is not implanted in the cell membrane. The β2m gene is located outside the MHC, on chromosome 15. The heavy chain is made up of three extramembrane domains, α1, α2 and α3. Each domain includes about 90 amino acids. Domains α2, α3 and β2m are stabilized by a disulphide bond. An oligosaccharide (CHO) is bound to the asparagine 86 of the α1 domain.

The class II molecule is a heterodimer composed of a heavy chain α($\approx$32 kDa) and a light chain β($\approx$28 kDa). Each chain comprises two extramembrane domains. The difference in molecular weight between the two chains depends on their glyco sylation: one oligosaccharide on the β chain, and two on the α chain. An invariant, strongly glycosylated chain li (31 or 33 kDa) is associated with the α and β chains in the endoplasmic reticulum, then dissociates in the endolysosomal compartment. The N-terminal extremity of this transmembrane chain is intracytoplasmic; Ii is not expressed at the cell membrane. The Ii gene is located on chromosome 5.

genes, may have a functional relationship with the MHC. In contrast, certain molecules participating in the presentation function, such as β2 microglobulin (β2m), and the invariant chain (li), are encoded outside the MHC (Figures 3.2 and 3.3).

3.1 Variability and Polymorphism

High variability and polymorphism are characteristic of the MHC. They are related to the function of presentation molecules and responsible for

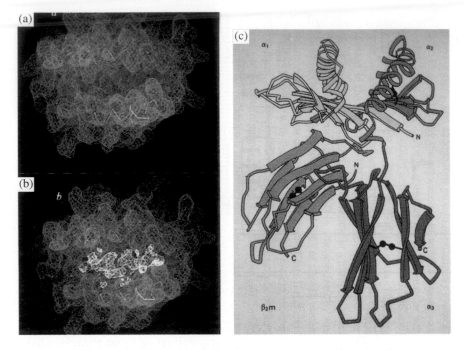

Figure 3.3 Three-dimensional structure of MHC1 molecule.

Schematic representation of the MHC1 molecule derived from the crystallo-graphic structure of HLA-A2 (from Bjorkman *et al.*,[3] with permission). (a) Top view of the α1 and α2 domains (van der Waals surface in blue). The α helices and the groove identified as the peptide binding site are shown. In (b) the groove is occupied by a peptide (pink) that co-purified and co-crystallized with HLA-A2. (c) Side view of the molecule showing the polymorphic α1 and α2 domains at the top and the α3 and β2m immunoglobulin like domains at the bottom. The spheres represent disulphide bonds. (Copyright © 1987 Macmillan Magazines Ltd.)

The homology of class II and class I sequences suggested a similar structure for both molecules. This was confirmed by X-ray crystallographic analysis of the HLA-DR1 molecule.

histoincompatibility phenomena. Variability is defined by the degree of difference between two allele genes and their products, measured by the number of different nucleotides or amino acids. Polymorphism is defined in a population by the number and frequencies of alleles at a locus.

Variable residues of the MHC1 molecule are mostly located in the α1 and α2 domains. Two alleles may differ by as many as 30 residues. Variability is high and mainly located at the functional site of the molecule: the presentation groove of the peptide and the contact region with TCR (α-helices). A comparable distribution of variable residues is observed for class II molecules. However, part of the functional site is invariable (DRα1) or little variable (DQα1 and DPα1). Variability is above all concentrated in the β1 domain of the β chain. The HLA Dictionary 2004[4] lists more than 1,300 alleles at the HLA-A, B, Cw, DR, DQ and DP loci.

MHC1 molecules contribute to the immune surveillance of the cell membrane. Peptides derived from viral or tumour proteins synthesized by the cell are presented at the cell membrane by MHC1 molecules. The complex is then recognized as non-self by the T cell repertoire, and the cells displaying the peptides are destroyed by cytotoxic T lymphocytes. During the process, the CD8 co-receptor interacts with the α3 domain of the MHC1 molecule.

MHC2 molecules mainly present to TCR peptides derived from extracellular or membrane proteins. The proteins are introduced into the cell via the endosomal route (Figure 3.4). The extracellular origin of these peptides has been demonstrated in many xenogeneic protein immunization protocols. CD4+ T lymphocytes obtained after immunization proliferate *in vitro* in the presence of the immunizing protein. However, this protein must be processed by antigen-presenting cells; the latter may be professional (macrophage, B cell), expressing MHC2 molecules constitutively, or occasional, bearing induced MHC2. During the interaction of the MHC2-peptide complex with the TCR, the CD4 co-receptor binds to the β2 domain of the MHC2 molecule. The immune response of CD4+ (helper) T lymphocytes is accompanied by the secretion of lymphokines, delayed hypersensitivity reaction, and contribute to the humoral response through T–B cell cooperation.

In addition to their antigen-presenting function during the immune response, MHC molecules also play a major role in the acquisition of the T lymphocyte repertoire. Hematopoietic stem cells from the bone marrow differentiate into T lymphocytes in the thymus on contact with MHC molecules. The thymus comprises a cortical zone containing epithelial cells and a medullary zone containing both epithelial cells and cells of hematopoietic origin. All these cells express MHC1 and 2 molecules in large quantities. T cell maturation occurs during their progression through the thymus from

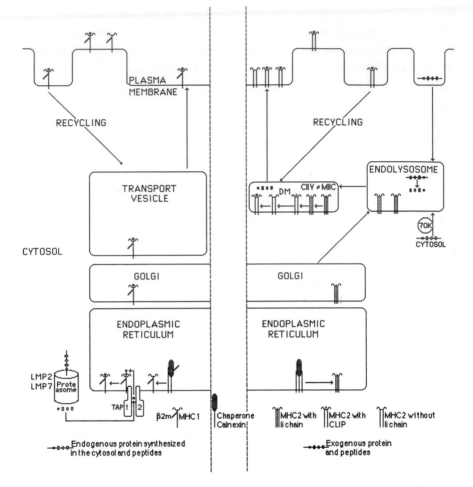

Figure 3.4 Endogenous (cytosolic) and exogenous (endosomal) pathways for peptide presentation by class I and class II MHC molecules.

The left-hand side of the figure represents the endogenous pathway. Class I molecules are synthesized in the endoplasmic reticulum (ER). The folding and assembly of the molecule may be controlled by a chaperone protein, calnexin. Peptide binding follows the assembly of the α chain and of β2m. The endogenous protein is principally synthesized in the cytosol. It may be degraded into peptides by the proteasome, of which at least two elements (LMP2 and LMP7) are coded in the MHC. Peptide transport in the ER may be achieved via the peptide pump composed of two elements (TAP1 and TAP2) coded in the MHC and inserted in the ER membrane. Peptides may enter the ER by other, unspecified paths. They may bind the cortical to the medullary zone. During this transit, the T cells multiply and, by a random rearrangement of their genes, generate a large number of TCRs. The T cells are then selected in function of the specificity of their TCR. The MHC thus permits the immune system to distinguish between

---

Figure 3.4 (*Continued*)

directly to the MHC1 molecule, or after concentration by chaperone molecules. Some peptides derive from proteins synthesized in the ER. The MHC1+peptide complex crosses the compartments of the Golgi apparatus and then reaches the cell membrane in a transport vesicle.

When β2m associates with class I heavy chain, calnexin dissociates and MHC1 becomes part of a peptide loading complex comprising TAP, tapasin, calreticulin and another chaperone protein ERp57. Tapasin plays a key role in shaping the MHC1 peptide repertoire.

The exogenous route (on the right) is characterized by the encounter in a specialized compartment (MHC class II compartment: MIIC; or class II-containing vesicle: CIIV) of MHC2 molecules and exogenous or membrane proteins. Class II α, β and Ii chains are synthesized and assembled (possibly with the aid of a chaperone protein) in the ER. The $\alpha\beta$Ii trimer, in the $(\alpha\beta$Ii)3 form, is transported through the compartments of the Golgi apparatus towards an endolysosome containing proteins endocytosed by the cell. During the transport the Ii chain is partially proteolyzed but a Ii fragment (class II-associated invariant-chain peptide: CLIP) is left in the MHC2 groove. In the specialized compartment the DM and DO molecules contribute to the replacement of CLIP by the endocytosed peptides. Endogenous cytosolic proteins may also be transferred into the endoiysosome by a process dependent upon a heat shock 70 kDa protein. A pH gradient (5–7) permits proteolysis and the dissociation of the chain, and the proteolysis and binding of (mostly) exogenous peptides.

At the cell surface, most MHC1 and MHC2 molecules carry a bound peptide, but a few "empty" molecules are probably present at the membrane. Mature MHC1 and MHC2 molecules of the plasma membrane may be internalized and recycled towards the membrane after passage in an endosomal compartment where they may bind a new peptide. Because of distinct assembly routes for MHC1 and MHC2 molecules, and because of the presence of the Ii chain, each molecule is specialized in the presentation of an endogenous or exogenous peptide, respectively; exceptions do, however, exist.

the self and the non-self, by contributing to the generation of a T cell repertoire capable of recognizing the self MHC presenting a non-self peptide.
The tolerance of self peptides is necessary to prevent self-destruction in the
organism by the immune system. This is usually a negative phenomenon:
non-recognition of self peptides by counter-selection of the appropriate
TCR (Table 3.1).

Table 3.1 Comparison of the properties and characteristics of MHC1 and MHC2
molecules.

	MHC1	MHC2
Expression	On practically all nucleated cells	On APC[a] and B lymphocytes, endothelial cells
T lymphocyte	100,000 mol./cell	Not expressed[b]
B lymphocyte	260,000 mol./cell	80,000 mol./cell[c]
Synthesis and expression time[d]	≈1 hour	≈3 hours
Renewal time ($t_{1/2}$) at the cell membrane[e]	8–10 hours	36 hours
Associated peptide	8–9 residues of cytosolic origin	13–30 residues of extra-cellular or membrane origin
T lymphocyte recognizing the MHC-peptide complex and consequences	CD8*, cytotoxic: target lysis	CD4+, helper, T cell proliferation: T–B cooperation and B cell response

[a] Antigen-presenting cells: monocyte-macrophages, dendritic cells of the skin,
lymph nodes and thymus. Thymic epithelium.
[b] A small number of activated T lymphocytes (<5% of circulating T lymphocytes)
express MHC2 molecules.
[c] DR molecules are more numerous than DQ and DP molecules.
[d] Time elapsing between synthesis in the endoplasmic reticulum and expression at
the cell membrane.
[e] Time necessary for replacement of half the molecules at the membrane by newly
synthesized molecules. A fraction of the molecules may be internalized and recycled.

3.2 Importance of HLA Compatibility in Transplantation

Transplantation is a standard treatment for several fatal diseases. Graft rejection is due to an immune response to MHC and minor antigens. It is necessary for donors and recipients to be HLA-identical in bone marrow transplantation (BMT) and in kidney transplantation. The best results are obtained when donor and recipient are HLA-identical siblings. On the other hand, heart and liver transplantations are performed in most cases in the situation of HLA incompatibility with fair results, because of efficient immunosuppression. One has thus to ask the question of the utility of HLA matching for kidney transplantation from cadaver-donor. Organizations have been developed for the distribution of cadaver-donor kidney transplants to patients awaiting transplantation. HLA compatibility is a factor among others for the choice of the recipient on the waiting list. Its relative importance is still discussed after 40 years of kidney transplantation practice. Another question is raised by the high and still growing number of alleles at the main HLA-A, B, DRB1 and DQB1 loci. Such a degree of polymorphism makes very difficult an HLA compatibility between donor and recipient when they are unrelated. Simplified HLA typing can then be used (Table 3.2).

Several studies show a significant role of HLA compatibility when cadaver-donor kidneys are transplanted to recipients under efficient immunosuppression (cyclosporine A). HLA compatibility is an important factor for long-term (10–20 years) graft survival, a particularly relevant issue considering the shortage of organs available for transplantation (Table 3.3). In practice a first choice is made after low-resolution HLA-A, B and DR typing, then allele matching is done whenever possible. Priority being given to zero A, B, DR mismatch, mismatches are then accepted at A, B and DR loci, in that order. Permissible mismatches will be preferred. Currently an identification of permissible versus immunogenic mismatches is being done by comparing mismatches in long surviving (more than seven years) versus rejected incompatible grafts.[5] Beside compatibility, choice of the recipient has to take into account the waiting time and the urgency of the transplantation.

For BMT, HLA identity between donor and recipient is necessary, but only about 30% of patients who need a BMT have an HLA-identical sibling.

Table 3.2 HLA typing for clinical purpose.

Because of the number of alleles, routine HLA typing cannot be exhaustive. Initially HLA typing was done by serological technique (microlymphocytotoxicity). Serology is currently being replaced by molecular biology techniques, but is still necessary for antibody screening in patients awaiting transplantation, and for pre-transplant crossmatch. Specificities originally defined by serology are often subdivided into several alleles (up to 70 in some instances). Most of the serological specificities form a family of alleles, with one allele predominant in a given population (Caucasian, black or Asiatic). The probable allele can thus be determined.

(a)	(b)	(c)	(d)
HLA-A	21	262	48
HLA-B	46	478	104
HLA-Cw	14	116	32
HLA-DRB1	15	300	65
HLA-DRB3,4,5	8	54	10
HLA-DQB1	9	43	20
HLA-DPB1	>63	>100	32

(a) HLA locus; (b) number of specificities or group of specificities; (c) number of alleles defined by DNA technologies and/or serological methods; (d) number of most frequent specificities usually determined for matching in transplantation.[4]

For that reason more than six million unrelated donors have been made available through worldwide programmes. HLA-DRBl and DQB1 typing must be as exhaustive as possible. The probability of finding an HLA identical donor rests on the HLA genotype of the recipient; patients carrying conserved and frequent haplotypes are naturally favoured, as well as patients of European-Caucasian descent, the population most represented in the donor files. Thanks to improved HLA typing techniques, results of BMT from unrelated donors are now comparable to those from HLA identical siblings.

MHC molecules participate in the immune response together with TCR, B cell receptor and antibodies. Polymorphism of MHC molecules is a consequence of their function of peptide presentation. Then polymorphism is responsible for the allogeneic response after transplantation. Compatibility is thus an important factor for the success of transplantation. Progress is being made toward induction of specific tolerance to the graft instead of permanent immunosuppression. The immune system discriminates between self

Table 3.3 Importance of HLA matching on graft survival.

(a)	0	1	2	3	4	5	6
(b)	40%	24%	20%	18%	17%	15%	13%

Notes: Graft survival (b) at 20 years post-transplantation in patients receiving first cadaver-donor kidney transplant, with 0-6 HLA-A, B, DR mismatches (a).[5]

Opelz *et al.* performed a collaborative study on 150,000 recipients transplanted from 1987 to 1997. They found a significant effect of HLA matching on graft and patient survival in kidney transplants (P < 0.0001). Graft survival rate at 10 years was 17% lower for transplants with 6 HLA−A+B+DR mismatches than that of transplants with no mismatch. For heart transplants, a significant impact of HLA compatibility was observed (P < 0.0001), but none for liver transplants.[6]

Claas *et al.* found that organ selection for highly immunized patients is based on complete compatibility with the patient's own HLA antigens (negative crossmatch), eventually in combination with acceptable mismatches. Specificities absent from the patient's HLA type without any reactive antibody are determined after extensive screening, in the patient's serum.[7]

and non-self, establishing unresponsiveness to self (self-tolerance). Immune response to alloantigens represents the main obstacle to allotransplantation. To establish graft tolerance on the model of self-tolerance would be the ideal for organ transplantation.[8] The characterization of regulatory T cells (Treg : $CD4^+$, $CD25^+$) in the context of self-tolerance suggests the possibility of using them for induction of graft tolerance. Pre-transplant blood transfusions have been shown to improve organ allograft survival. Induction of $CD4^+$ Treg may at least in part, account for the beneficial effect of these transfusions. Transfusions sharing at least one HLA-DR with the recipient are more effective than HLA-mismatched transfusions. Treg recognizing an allopeptide in the context of self HLA-DR would be generated before the transplantation.[9] Studies on how to control immunoregulatory cells would provide a complementary approach to preventing T cell activation (HLA compatibility + immunosuppression).

References

1. Chen, X and Jensen, P.E. (2004). The Expression of HLA-DO (H2-O) in B Lymphocytes, *Immunol Res*, **29**, 19–28.

2. Herberg, J.A., Beck, S. and Trowsdale, J. (1998). TAPASIN, DAXX, RGL2, HKE2 and Four New Genes (BING 1, 3 to 5) Form a Dense Cluster at the Centromeric End of the MHC, *J Mol B*, **277**, 839–857.
3. Bjorkman, P.J. *et al.* (1987). Structure of the Human Class I Histocompatibility Antigen, HLA-A2, *Nature*, **329**, 506–512.
4. Schreuder, G.M. *et al.* (2005). HLA Dictionary 2004: Summary of HLA-A, -B, -C, -DRB1/3/4/5, -DQB1 Alleles and Their Association with Serologically Defined HLA-A, -B, -C, -DR, and -DQ Antigens, *Hum Immunol*, **66**, 170–210.
5. Terasaki, P.I. *et al.* (1995). Advances in Kidney Transplantation: 1985–1995, *Clin Transplant*, pp. 487–501.
6. Opelz, G. *et al.* (1999). HLA Compatibility and Organ Transplant Survival. Collaborative Transplant Study, *Rev Immunogenet*, **1**, 334–342.
7. Claas, F.H. *et al.* (1999). Acceptable HLA Mismatches for Highly Immunized Patients, *Rev lmmunogenet*, **1**, 351–358.
8. Sakaguchi, S. (2004). Naturally Arising CD4+ Regulatory T Cells For Immunologic Self-tolerance and Negative Control of Immune Responses, *Annu Rev Immunol*, **22**, 531–562.
9. Roelen, D., Brand, A. and Claas, F.H. (2004). Pre-Transplant Blood Transfusions Revisited: A Role for CD(4+) Regulatory T Cells? *Transplantation*, **77(1 Suppl)**, S26–S28.

4

Skin Transplantation

Shahid A. Khan, John R. C. Telfer and Dai M. Davies

The skin is the largest single organ in the human body. It is a complex, bilayered structure that covers the body and isolates it from the surrounding environment. It is necessary for the homeostasis of the internal milieu and paramount in the defence against hostile environmental influences. The skin is the interface with the external environment and can induce an immune response defence and reject strange antigens. Small wounds with skin loss, if untreated, heal by secondary intention, with wound contraction and epithelialisation. This process may be associated with desiccation and necrosis of the underlying structures and wound contractures resulting in impairment of function. Conditions with significant skin loss lead to depletion of water, electrolytes and protein and the removal of an effective barrier to the entrance of bacteria and so are potentially life- threatening. In such circumstances skin cover may be lifesaving.

The commonest type of injury that destroys large areas of skin is a burn. The majority of burns which need skin cover are readily managed with autologous split skin grafts. However, a burn of greater than 30% total body surface area represents a significant challenge to the patient's own donor sites to meet the requirements for split skin grafts, although the use of meshing greatly extends the possible area that can be covered. A burn that covers over

70% of the body surface area may be too extensive to cover with autologous skin in a single procedure, although repeated harvesting of healed donor sites is possible. In certain circumstances there is therefore a requirement for skin that cannot be met by the patient's own resources.

4.1 Alternative Skin Cover

The need to replace skin loss has been recognised since the last century. Pollock advocated the value of early skin cover to relieve suffering, prevent contractures and avoid deformity. He is attributed with popularising the technique of skin grafting, first described by Reverdin, and with being the first to use allograft for a burn patient in 1870.[1] Girdner published on the use of cadaver skin for the treatment of burns in 1881 and at that time its use was regarded as a permanent solution.[2] Skin from a variety of different animals, including pigs and sheep, was also used with the same expectation. Only later was it recognised that autografts behaved in a different way to allografts. Brown and McDowell advocated the use of allografts as lifesaving in large burns, but noted: 'Homografts ... survive from three to ten weeks ... then absorb in a rather clean way'.[3] It was the increase in the rate of wound healing that caused some workers to believe that allografts took permanently. In 1943 Gibson and Medawar published the results of the first controlled experiments on the fate of skin allografts in humans. This work, which defined immunologic rejection and laid down many of the principles of immunology, such as the second set phenomenon, stands as a landmark in the development of transplant immunology.[4]

4.2 Allograft Skin

Allograft skin applied to a suitable wound bed will adhere and become vascularised in the same way as an autograft. Allograft skin is, however, strongly immunogenic and, ten days or more following application of the allograft skin, the process of rejection, leading to necrosis and separation of the donor skin, becomes clinically apparent. Further allografts from the same donor will be rejected more quickly.[4] Despite the problem of rejection, allograft skin has been shown to be of a considerable benefit, clinically.

It has been used in several different ways:

(a) as a biological dressing
(b) as temporary skin cover prior to definitive cover
(c) as definitive skin cover.

4.2.1 Allograft skin as a biological dressing

Allograft skin used as a biological dressing fulfils several functions:

(a) to reduce or prevent the appearance of granulation tissue
(b) to decrease bacterial counts in granulation tissue
(c) as a barrier to reduce the loss of fluid and protein
(d) to decrease pain
(e) to increase mobility
(f) to enhance the growth of autologous epithelium.[5,6]

To avoid the rejection response and necrosis of the recipient wound bed the allografts need to be changed every three days, as after this time they become firmly adherent, and removal is painful and causes bleeding.

Alternatively, the allografts may be left *in situ* until they are rejected. Brown and McDowell noted an improvement in the general condition of burns patients with the use of allograft skin. In addition, there was a stimulus to the patient's own epithelialisation such that wound healing could occur despite absorption of the allografts.[3] Jackson found that using alternate strips of autograft and allograft encouraged healing of the wound, even in the presence of allograft loss.[7]

4.2.2 Allograft skin as temporary skin cover

A significant burn will reduce the immunity of the patient to a certain degree but not sufficiently to usefully prolong allograft survival. Reported cases where allograft has survived for longer than expected have been attributed to multiple blood transfusions altering the immune system. However, in order to prolong survival of the allograft, predictably, either depression of the immune system itself or reduction of the antigenicity of the allograft is required.

The Langerhans cells, which are probably derived from the granulocyte-monocyte precursor line, express HLA–D/Dr antigens and may be involved in the initiation of a T-lymphocyte-dependent immune response, as seen in allograft rejection. Depletion of Langerhans cells in the allograft by ultra-violet irradiation and glucocorticoid treatment demonstrated some prolongation of allograft survival in seven patients but the range was large (22–96 days).[8] The failure to produce reliable long-term survival is attributed to invasion of host Langerhans cells into the allograft within a few days.

Depression of the immune system itself, as practiced in recipients of other allograft organs, has also been investigated. Initial studies using azathioprine demonstrated prolongation of survival of allograft skin.[9] Antithymocyte globulin showed a similar effect, but with a reduction in the incidence of leucopenia.[10] In these cases the allografts were serially excised and replaced by autografts, as sufficient quantities became available. Immunosuppression was continued until less than 20% of the total body surface area was still covered with allograft — up to 50 days. Withdrawal of immunosuppression led to clinical evidence of rejection of the remaining allograft some ten days later.

There was considerable concern about the difficulty of avoiding excessive immunosuppression with azathioprine in burns patients, who are particularly susceptible to infection. Borel showed that Cyclosporine A provided a more specific immunosuppression of the cell-mediated immune system, without the same risk of sepsis from depression of the bone marrow.[11] Further studies using Cyclosporine A have demonstrated survival of allograft skin until its withdrawal.[12,13] Little toxicity related to the use of Cyclosporine A has been demonstrated and any depression in the white-cell count has been rapidly reversed by withholding the Cyclosporine for a short period. Clinical studies of long-term survival remain largely experimental.[14] There have been isolated reports of transmission of viral infections from allografts skin whilst on Cyclosporine.[15] Cyclosporine A is not routinely used in burns today, but it may still have a place in the management of the occasional patient with a major burn, to buy time when autologous skin is scarce.[16]

4.2.3 Allograft skin for definitive skin cover

Various techniques have been developed to provide long-term, permanent skin cover. The use of widely meshed autograft skin covered with less widely meshed allograft skin has been advocated as a way of promoting permanent healing of large burn wounds.[17] Using this technique, Phipps and Clarke found no clinically appreciable rejection of the allograft skin. The use of biotinylated probe specific for the Y chromosome in one patient, however, suggested that the allograft skin probably does not survive long term; rather, autograft cells replace it by a process of creeping substitution.[18]

The benefit of the allograft skin to provide prompt wound cover and provide a suitable environment for survival and propagation of the scanty autograft is clear: providing a biological dressing to inhibit granulation tissue formation whilst epithlialisation occurs, it allows a transition from intermingled skin grafts to healed wound without the need for a secondary procedure, thus reducing the chance of subsequent graft contracture. The technique was used mainly in children and the donor was usually a parent, providing readily available fresh allograft and reducing the likelihood of unsuspected viral transmission from donor to recipient.

Anatomically, dermis constitutes 95% of skin and provides foundation for epidermis. From clinical experience, burns surgeons have come to appreciate that preservation of the recipient dermis or transfer of a significant thickness of donor dermis in a skin graft, improves the durability for the graft during transfer, reduces the degree of contraction of the wound, and improves the quality and texture of the final wound cover. It has been speculated that the acellular components are more important in influencing graft development.[19] Studies using cultured kertinocytes have demonstrated better take and a more stable epithelium when the cultured sheets are placed on dermis rather than subcutaneous tissue.[20,21]

Medawar demonstrated the persistence of allogenic dermis, denuded of its epidermis but covered by host epidermis, and concluded that the dermis itself is less immunoreactive than the epidermis.[22] This suggests that the dermal support for the final epithelium need not be the host's.

Cuono modified a technique advocated by Heck.[23–25] Allograft skin is used to provide the initial skin cover but the allograft epidermis is removed by dermabrasian prior to rejection. The allograft dermis which is left behind appears less antigenic and provides a suitable bed for application of autograft split skin or cultured autokeratinocytes. It is not clear what becomes of the cellular elements of the allograft dermis, but it is likely that they are gradually replaced by the host cells. Cuono felt that the reappearance of anchoring fibrils and the rapidly orderly stratification and maturation of the cultured keratinocytes into differentiated mature epidermis, was evidence for a functioning dermis. The noncellular component of the dermis survives, albeit in a modified form, and it may be this that contributes significantly to the quality of the scarring in the long term and to the adherence of the epidermis.[26]

Wainwright has investigated the use of an acellular allograft dermal matrix (Alloderm) to provide 'a non-immunogenic template' to augment the dermal support for widely meshed split-thickness autografts.[27] Wendt proved that it is possible for human skin allografts to survive indefinitely on patients taking the usual dosages of immunosuppressants used for renal transplantation.[28] In his study of six patients, Wendt observed that there was minimal repopulation of skin allografts by autogenous keratinocytes and fibroblast while patients were taking immunosuppressants. When immuno-suppression was discontinued in two patients after six weeks and five years (respectively) due to renal transplant rejection, Wendt observed that the skin allograft cells were destroyed and replaced with autogenous cells, but the skin graft did not reject acutely and persisted clinically. Based on these observations Wendt hypothesised that the acellular portion of the skin allograft was not rejected acutely because of relatively low antigenicity and because it acted as a lattice for autogenous cells to migrate into and replace rejected allograft skin cells. No chimerism was seen in autogenous skin in the skin–renal transplant patients in the study.[28]

4.2.4 Sources of allograft skin

Allograft skin is widely used in burns units today, but concerns about the transmission of bacterial and viral infections, particularly the human immunodeficiency virus (HIV), have restricted the routine use of allograft skin, to those with major burns.[29] The screening of donors and the use of living-related donors should minimise the risk.

However, neither fresh donor cadavers nor living-related donors are always readily available. This has led to the development of skin banks and techniques to store skin. Initially, allografts were treated with 0.5% glutaraldehyde and stored at 4°C, but this led to early deterioration characterised by epidermolysis. The use of glycerol in high concentration (85%)

to preserve skin was introduced in 1983 and has been used as the method of choice in many centres. Modern cryopreservation techniques use 30% glycerol or 5% DMSO as cryoprotective agents. The graft is freeze-dried and stored for use for up to seven years. Glycerol preserves skin structure as it replaces water extracted from the cells and distributes the remaining water throughout the tissue. Moreover, glycerol does not affect the collagen and elastin fibres present in the dermis. Glycerol-preserved allografts have better primary adherence by fibrin bonding and secondary adherence by fibrovascular in growth. In addition, glycerol reduces the antigenicity of tissues used in transplantation.[30] Glycerol also has an effective bateriostatic and antiviral action. Some pathogens can be eliminated, without significantly affecting skin structure, through additional radiation sterilisation process.

Freeze-drying allograft skin is the preservation method preferred by many centres, due to its superior physiological properties. However, it requires specialised storage and rapid thawing facilities, which complicates its use.

4.2.5 Artificial skin

There has been no success in finding a substitute for autograft skin which has texture and function like natural skin, is readily available and low cost, has no antigenicity, and has rapid and sustained adherence to the wound surface to provide immediate definitive wound cover. However, there are a number of tissue-engineered products available commercially which are being used as temporary and long-term wound cover.

4.2.5.1 *Cellular skin substitutes*

The use of cultured autograft keratinocytes (Epicel: Genzyme Tissue Repair, Cambridge, MA) requires an initial small skin-biopsy specimen, approximately three weeks to grow the keratinocyte grafts in culture, and the use of a dermal substitute to stabilise the cultured epidermal layer. Although cosmetically acceptable results are possible, the use of such a skin substitute is costly and requires time. Cultured keratinocyte allografts obviate the initial biopsy and the time involved in culturing the graft, but they are also expensive and may lead to disease transmission.[31]

4.2.5.2 *Acellular skin substitutes*

Several options for artificial dermal graft skin substitutes exist. These include bovine collagen and chondroitin-6-sulfate over silicone (Integra: Integra LifeSciences, Plainsboro, NJ), and fibroblast nylon or bioabsorbable mesh (Dermagraft: Advanced Tissue Sciences Inc., La Jolla, CA). Intregra is currently the most commonly used skin substitute. Despite the immediate availability of acellular skin substitutes, their expense and potential for disease transmission in the case of allograft-derived dermal grafts limits their usefulness.[31]

Apligraf (Organogenis, Canton, MA) (a bioengineered, bilayered skin equivalent composed of bovine type I collagen, allogeneic human skin fibroblasts, and cultured neonatal foreskin-derived keratinocytes) functions as an effective skin substitute. Although it is currently Food and Drug Administration (FDA) approved for use in the treatment of venous ulcers, ongoing studies are being conducted to investigate its effectiveness in the treatment of cutaneous surgical defects.

Another living skin equivalent, composite cultured skin (OrCel), consists of allogeneic fibroblasts and keratinocytes seeded on opposite sides of a bilayered matrix of bovine collagen. There are limited clinical data available for this product. Limited data are also available for two types of dressing material derived from pigs: porcine small intestinal submucosa acellular collagen matrix (Oasis) and an acellular xenogeneic collagen matrix (E-Z-Derm).

Other novel skin substitutes are being investigated. The potential risks and benefits of using tissue-engineered skin need to be further evaluated in clinical trials but it is obvious that they offer a new option for the treatment of wounds.

4.3 Transplant of Composite Tissues Involving Skin

The advances in the microvascular techniques and development of effective immunosuppressive drugs have enabled reconstructive surgeons to successfully transplant composite human tissue. Hand transplantation was first performed in 1998 and acceptable functional and cosmetic outcomes have been claimed. The active range of motion of the digits has been much better than expected, and a considerable improvement on the results of previous replantations. However, the return of sensibility has been less than optimal. The immunosuppression has been well tolerated, but some patients have developed chronic viral and fungal infections and several have developed post-transplant diabetes.[32] However, the hand transplant recipient requires lifelong immunosupression with a high risk of getting a life-threatening infection, and normal return of two-point discrimination or intrinsic muscle function, both necessary for fine motor use, is not to be expected. Furthermore, the effects of chronic rejection on the allograft function and survival have not yet been determined. Preliminary clinical experience in hand transplant has underscored the importance of patient motivation and compliance, intensive hand therapy, and close post-transplantation surveillance. In summary, hand transplantation is a procedure that enhances the function and appearance of carefully selected patients. Further research and progress in transplant immunology are needed before it can be considered a consistently safe and efficacious practice.

4.4 The Future

The replantation of an avulsed whole face on a girl in India, reported almost ten years ago, has offered new hope for reconstruction of facial burns, extensive malignancy and trauma. Long-term survival of a transplanted face in the rat model was achieved, without any signs of rejection, with low-dose immunosuppressive therapy.[33] Some do not doubt a face will be transferred from a corpse to a living human, believing it is only a question of when and where. The question of long-term survival is a major concern in human face transplantation.

For the reconstructive surgeon, the major challenge remains skin cover of major burns. Modulation of the antigenicity of the allograft and refinements in the long-term immunosuppression of the recipient would be significant advances in the use of allograft skin. Further development of bioengineered allogenic cellular dermis combined with cultured allokeratinocytes, may provide a truly immediately available, permanent skin cover. As the development of these new techniques advances they may be applied in many situations: to provide skin cover following excision of giant congenital naevii or extensive skin malignancies; to cover major degloving injuries; to remove the extra morbidity associated with skin graft donor sites. Perhaps the need of autologous skin, one of the greatest problems in plastic surgery, may be permanently removed.

Advances in bio-technologically developed human parts, and transplant of these composite tissues, would enable reconstructive surgeons to offer the ultimate reconstruction, replacing like with like. Professor Jean-Michel Dubernard led the world's first face transplant in France on 27 November 2005. The 38-year-old female recipient, who had been disfigured in a dog attack, received a new nose, lips and chin from a donor (*The Times*, 2005).

References

1. Freshwater, M.F. and Krizek, T.J. (1978). George David Pollock and the Development of Skin Grafting, *Ann Plas Surg*, **1**, 96–102.
2. Girdner, J.H. (1881). Skin Grafting with Grafts Taken from the Dead Subject, *Med Rec*, **20**, 119–120.
3. Brown, J.B. and McDowell, F. (1942). Massive Repairs of Burns with Thick Split Skin Grafts, *Ann Surg*, **115**, 658–674.
4. Gibson, T. and Medawar, P.B. (1943). The Fate of Skin Homografts in Man, *J Anat*, **77**, 299–310.
5. Artz, C.P. *et al.* (1972). An Appraisal of Allografts and Xenografts as Biological Dressings for Wounds and Burns, *Ann Surg* **175**, 934–938.
6. Alsbjorn, B. (1984). In Search of an Ideal Skin Substitute, *Scand J Plastic Recons*, **18**, 127–133.
7. Jackson, D. (1954). A Clinical Study for the Use of Skin Homografts for Burns, *Brit J Plas Surg*, **7**, 26–43.
8. Alsbjorn, B. and Sorenson, B. (1985). Grafting with Epidermal Langerhans Cell Depressed Cadaver Skin, *Burns*, **11**, 259–263.
9. Burke, J.F. *et al.* (1974). Temporary Skin Transplantation and Immunosuppression for Extensive Burns, *New Engl J Med*, **290**, 269–271.
10. Burke, J.F. *et al.* (1975). Immunosupression and Temporary Skin Transplantation in the Treatment of Massive Third-Degree Burns, *Ann Surg*, **182**, 183–197.
11. Borel, J.F. *et al.* (1977). Effects of the New Anti-Lymphocytic Peptides Cyclosporine A in Animals, *Immunology*, **32**, 1017–1025.
12. Achauer, B.M. *et al.* (1986). Long-Term Skin Allograft after Short-Term Cyclosporine Treatment in a Patient with Massive Burns, *Lancet*, **1**, 14–15.
13. Frame, J.D. *et al.* (1989). The Fate of Meshed Allograft Skin in Burned Patients Using Cyclosporine Immunosuppression, *Brit J Plast Surg*, **42**, 27–34.
14. Wendt, J.R. *et al.* (1994). Indefinite Survival of Human Skin Allografts in Patients With Long-Term Immunosupression, *Ann Plas Surg*, **32**, 411–417.

15. Bale, J.F. *et al.* (1991). Cytomegalovirus Infection in a Cyclosporine-Treated Burns Patient (Case Report), *J Traum*, **32**, 263–267.

16. Achauer, B.M. (1996). Personal Communication.

17. Alexander, J.W. *et al.* (1981). Treatment of Serve Burns with Widely Meshed Skin Autograft and Meshed Allograft Overlay, *J Traum*, **21**, 433–438.

18. Phipps, A.R. and Clarke, J.A. (1991). The Use of Intermingled Autograft and Parental Allograft Skin in the Treatment of Major Burns in Children, *Brit J Plast Surg*, **44**, 608–611.

19. MacNeil, S. (1994). What Role Does the Extra Cellularmatrix Serve in Skin Grafting and Wound Healing? *Burns*, **20**, s27–s70.

20. Eldad, A. *et al.* (1987). Cultured Epithelium as a Skin Substitute, *Burns*, **13**, 173–180.

21. Navsaria, H.A. *et al.* (1994). An Animal Model to Study the Significance of Dermis for Grafting Cultured Keratinocytes on Full Thickness Wounds, *Burns*, **20**, s57–s60.

22. Medawar, P.B. (1945). A Second Study of the Behaviour and Fate of Skin Homografts in Rabbits, *J Anat*, **79**, 157–176.

23. Cuono, C. *et al.* (1986). Use of Cultured Epidermal Allografts as Skin Replacement after Burn Injury, *Lancet*, **1**, 1123–1124.

24. Cuono, C. *et al.* (1987). Composite Autologous-Allogenic Skin Replacements: Development and Clinical Application, *Plast Reconstr Surg*, **42**, 626–635.

25. Heck, E.L. *et al.* (1985). Composite Skin Graft: Frozen Dermal Allografts Support the Engraftment and Expansion of Autologous Epidermis, *J Traum*, **25**, 16–112.

26. Hickerson, W.J. *et al.* (1994). Cultured Epidermal Autografts and Allodermis Combination for Permanent Burn Wound Coverage, *Burns*, **20**, s52–s56.

27. Wainwright, D.J. (1995). Use of an Acellular Dermal Matrix (Alloderm) in the Management of Full Thickness Burns, *Burns*, **21**, 243–248.

28. Wendt, J.R. *et al.* (2004). Long-Term Survival of Human Skin Allografts in Patients with Immunosuppression, *Am J Plast Reconstr Surg*, **113(5)**, 1347–1354.

29. Clarke, J.A. (1987). HIV Transmission and Skin Grafts, *Lancet*, **i**, 983.

30. Hoekstra, M.J. *et al.* (1994). History of the Euro Skin Bank: The Innovation of Preservation Techniques, *Burns*, **20**, s43–s47.

31. Bello, Y.M. *et al.* (2002). Tissue-Engineered Skin. Current Status in Wound Healing, *Am J Clin Dermatol*, **2(5)**, 305–513, 2001. See also Comment in: *A J Clin Dermatol* **3(7)**, 507, author reply 507–508, 2002.

32. Jones, N.F. (2002). Concerns about Human Hand Transplantation in the 21st Century, *Am J Hand Surg*, **27(5)**, 771–787.

33. Ulusal, B.G. *et al.* (2003). A New Composite Facial and Scalp Transplantation Model in Rats, *J Plast Reconstr Surg*, **112(5)**, 1302–1311.

5

Renal Transplantation

Nicos Kessaris and Nadey S. Hakim

5.1 History

Yu Yu Voronoy, a Soviet surgeon, performed the first human kidney transplant in 1933.[1] The donor was a 60-year-old male who had died 6 hours beforehand from a head injury. The recipient, a 26-year-old female with renal failure secondary to mercuric chloride overdose, died two days later as the graft never functioned. This transplant was across different blood groups and was placed in the thigh.[1] After a few more unsuccessful attempts in the 1930s, Voronoy stopped.

The first successful live kidney transplant was between two identical twins. The donor nephrectomy was performed by J. Hartwell Harrison and the transplant by Joseph Murray on 23 December 1954 at the Peter Bent Brigham Hospital in Boston.[2,3] The recipient survived for nine years, without immunosuppression until the graft eventually failed due to recurrent glomerulonephritis.

Immunosuppression was introduced in the early 1960s following pioneering work performed by Sir Roy Calne in London and Boston as well as by Thomas Starzl in Denver.[4,5] This involved the use of azathioprine and steroids.[6] Polyclonal antibody preparations like ATG (antithymocyte globulin) were introduced in the mid 1970s.[7] These were used either as induction agents or to treat steroid-resistant rejection. Kidney transplant survival of one year during that era was about 50%. In the early 1980s, cyclosporine was introduced and kidney-graft patients' survival rate increased to more than 80% at one year.[8,9]

Tacrolimus was introduced in the late 1980s as an alternative to cyclosporine.[10] Early studies showed that the two drugs had similar graft survival rates but patients treated with tacrolimus had fewer episodes of rejection that were less severe.[11,12] Over the years, the patients with one-year kidney survival rate increased to more than 90%.[13-17]

5.2 Live Donor Renal Transplantation

Graft success after live donor kidney transplantation is superior to cadaveric renal transplantation. In a study from the US that assessed outcomes from 1988 to 1996, the half-life of kidneys from live donors increased to 21.6 years, and that from cadaveric donors increased to 13.8 years over the study period.[18] Over the last ten years there has been a significant increase in the number of live donor renal transplants in the world.[19-21] In the UK, the number of live transplants has trebled over the same period (Figure 5.1).

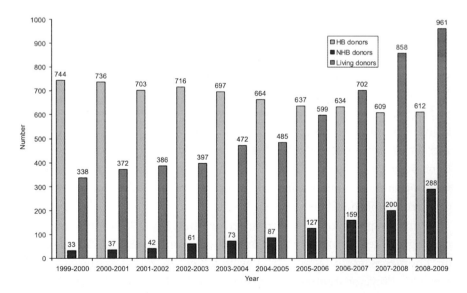

Figure 5.1 The total number of deceased and live donors in the UK between 1 April 1999 and 31 March 2009.[23] Including the living organ donors, there were 15 altruistic and 16 paired live kidney donors.

Between 1 April 2009 and 31 March 2010, there were 1,026 such transplants in the UK.[22]

A similar increase in live donor transplants was observed in the US until 2007. Since then there has been a slow reduction in the number of such transplants.[20] There are current attempts to reverse this downward trend through the increased use of laparoscopic donor nephrectomy, the finger-assisted nephrectomy, antibody incompatible transplantation, pair exchange programmes and economic support for donors.[20]

5.3 Live Donor Evaluation

In the UK potential donors are assessed according to standards and guidelines provided by the British Transplantation Society.[24] The evaluation includes past medical history and assessment of the psychosocial state. This is followed by an examination of the cardiac, respiratory and abdominal systems. Investigations include routine haematology and biochemistry, as well as virology. The latter includes tests for hepatitis B and C, cytomegalovirus, HIV-1 and HIV-2, and Epstein–Barr virus. Cardiovascular investigations include a chest X-ray, ECG and, where necessary, an exercise ECG and echocardiogram. At least three urine dipsticks are performed to check for haematuria. Samples are also sent for microscopy, culture and sensitivity. Ultrasonography assesses the size of the kidneys, and if there is more than 1 cm difference between the two kidneys, split function is assessed by combining an European Dialysis and Transplant Association glomerular filtration rate (EDTA GFR) with a dimercaptosuccinic acid (DMSA) scan. A computed tomography (CT) or magnetic resonance imaging (MRI) provides a way of assessing the number of renal arteries present in the donor.[25]

5.4 Donor Nephrectomy

There are a number of different ways of performing a donor nephrectomy. These are divided into the open approaches and the laparoscopic ones. The traditional open approach involves a 15 to 20 cm incision in the loin and is the most invasive out of all nephrectomy procedures.

The mini-open or finger-assisted donor nephrectomy involves a much smaller incision in the loin with much less morbidity. Dissection around

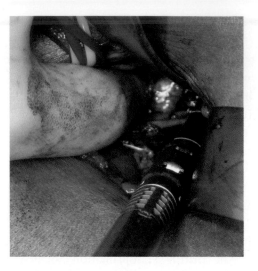

Figure 5.2 Showing the endoscopic linear cutter being used to divide the renal artery during a left mini-open donor nephrectomy.

the kidney is similar to the open procedure but includes a linear articulated stapling device (the ETS-Flex 35 mm, Articulating, Endoscopic Linear Cutter, manufactured by Ethicon Endo-Surgery, Inc., Cincinnati, OH) to divide the vessels. Retraction is maintained using two thin handheld wound retractors with a light source attached and the index and middle finger of the surgeon (see Figure 5.2). The main surgeon uses a headlight with magnification loupes.[26] Figure 5.3 shows the kidney removed with the finger-assisted technique.

There are pure laparoscopic approaches and hand-assisted ones. The first pure laparoscopic donor nephrectomy was performed by Ratner in 1995 at Johns Hopkins University's School of Medicine (Baltimore, MD, USA).[27] This procedure is more demanding than the hand-assisted approach, and involves the insertion of four ports.

The hand-assisted approach involves having one hand inside the abdomen during the procedure, through a lower midline or a Pfannenstiel incision. Two or three further small incisions are made to allow the insertion of a laparoscope attached to a video camera and the harmonic scalpel® (Ethicon Endo-Surgery, Inc., Cincinnati, OH) to perform the dissection around the kidney (Figure 5.4). Dissection can be transperitoneal[28] or retroperitoneal.[29,30] The former involves gaining access to the abdominal

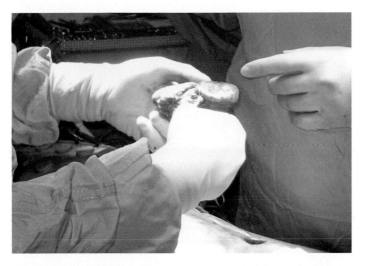

Figure 5.3 Showing the kidney having been extracted from a small loin incision.

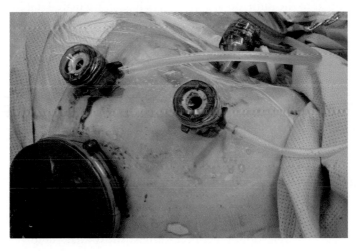

Figure 5.4 The GelPort® Hand Access Device (Applied Medical, Rancho Santa Margarita, CA) and three standard ports in preparation for a right-side retroperitoneal live donor nephrectomy.

cavity first, before reflecting the colon towards the middle to get to the kidney. The latter involves creating a space behind the peritoneum by reflecting it from the abdominal wall towards the middle. This avoids the mobilisation of the colon and other structures like the lower aspect of the

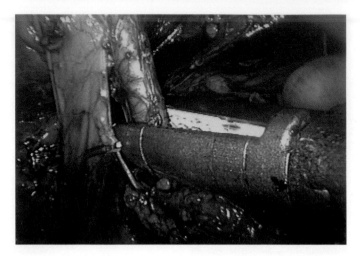

Figure 5.5 The endoscopic linear cutter used to staple and divide the renal artery.

spleen. Similar to the mini-open approach, a linear articulated stapling device (ETS-Flex 35 mm, Articulating, Endoscopic Linear Cutter) is used for dividing the vessels (Figure 5.5).

More recently, single-port techniques have been devised in the US[31] but these seem to be associated with longer, warm ischaemia times. A trans-vaginal approach has been used to retrieve live donor kidneys from female patients in the US and Spain.[32,33] Infection does not seem to be an issue in these initial series but long-term outcomes are still awaited.

5.5 Complications

Large single-centre studies, as well as large surveys reviewing hand-assisted and pure laparoscopic donor nephrectomies, show that these procedures are generally safe but that they require great attention.[34–39] Advantages over the traditional open operation include reduced post-operative pain and in-hospital stay as well as earlier return to work. A number of randomised clinical trials have also confirmed these advantages.[40–43]

A meta-analysis comparing pure laparoscopic versus hand-assisted live donor nephrectomy showed similar complication rates for both operations. The main difference between the two techniques was that the hand-assisted one was associated with less operative and warm ischaemic time as well as intraoperative bleeding.[44] Conversion to open procedure varies from 0.2%

to 2.8% but it becomes less with experience.[36] Severe bleeding is rare using laparoscopic approaches but can be fatal.[45]

A large UK review assessing donor outcomes between 2000 and 2006 showed the overall minor morbidity to be 14.3% and the major morbidity to be 4.9%.[39] Laparoscopic approaches had significantly less minor complications but similar major complications when compared to open techniques. A number of studies from the US have reported the risk of death to be 0.03%.[37,38] This has remained constant over the last 15 years.[38]

Longer-term complications stemming from any type of procedure include hypertension and proteinuria.[46,47] All donors should be called in for a yearly follow-up, for life.

5.6 Cadaveric Renal Transplantation

The number of patients waiting for cadaveric renal transplantation rises with time (Figure 5.6). There are currently 6,855 patients in the UK and 86,142 patients in the USA waiting for cadaveric renal transplantation.[48,49]

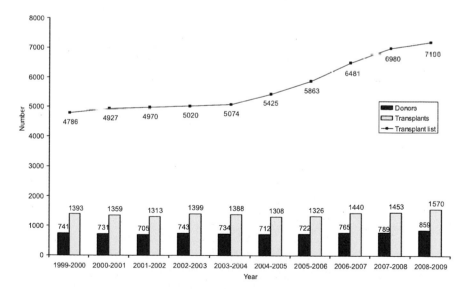

Figure 5.6 The number of patients waiting for cadaveric renal transplantation in the UK over the last ten years. This graph summarises the cadaveric renal transplant activity during the same period.[23] Activity includes heart-beating and non-heart-beating donor kidney transplants.

Cadaveric renal transplantation can be from either heart-beating or non-heart-beating donors. The latter is also known as donation after cardiac death. In the UK, the number of heart-beating donors was around 700 per year from 2000 to 2004. This number has decreased between 2005 and 2009 to around 600 donors per year. The number of non-heart-beating donors has doubled between 2007 and 2009 to around 300 such donors per year. These results are summarised in Figure 5.1. The total number of deceased donors has therefore increased as has the total number of renal transplants (Figure 5.6).[23]

5.7 Deceased Heart–Beating Donor (HBD)

In the UK there were 624 HBDs between April 2009 and April 2010, and 335 NHBDs during the same period. That comes to a total of 959 donors.[22] This is the highest number ever of cadaveric donors in one year in the UK.

5.8 Non–Heart–Beating Donor (NHBD)

NHBDs are classified according to the Maastricht classification of NHBD (Table 5.1). Another way of classifying NHBDs is as 'uncontrolled' (categories I, II) or 'controlled' (categories III, IV). This depends on whether cardiopulmonary function stops spontaneously or after withdrawal of medical therapy.[50,51]

Table 5.1 The Maastricht classification of non–heart–beating donors.[50,51]

Category	Type of potential donor
I	Dead on arrival
II	Unsuccessful resuscitation
III	Awaiting cardiac arrest
IV	Cardiac arrest in a brainstem-dead donor

Some 80% of kidneys come from NHBD experience-delayed graft function (DGF).[52] Patients with DGF will require dialysis until the kidney starts working, usually after a few days. If the kidney does not start working, the patient needs to have a biopsy at one week after transplantation to exclude rejection. DGF can be reduced using machine perfusion rather than cold storage to transfer the kidney for the donor to the recipient hospital.[53,54]

Over the last few years there have been two randomised controlled studies assessing the use of machine perfusion for non-heart-beating kidneys prior to transplantation. One was carried out in Europe and the other in the UK. The former[54] favoured its use and the latter[55] did not, with respect to reduction in DGF as well as one-year graft function.

Five-year graft survival and function from NHBDs are comparable to those from HBDs. But for retransplants or for when cold ischaemic time is more than 12 hours, the graft survival is worse.[52]

5.9 Renal Transplantation

5.9.1 Recipient evaluation

All recipients undergo a thorough history and examination including abdominal examination and examination of the full compliment of pulses in the legs. History includes assessment of cardiac risk factors including age greater than 50 years, angina, ischaemic heart disease, high cholesterol, diabetes, cerebrovascular disease, peripheral vascular disease, if the patient has been on dialysis for more than five years. Other aspects include urological history as well as history of cancer. Patients need to be disease free for up to five years after curative therapy for cancer.

Routine investigations include haematology, biochemistry and virology. The latter includes a hepatitis screen (B and C), CMV, HIV and EBV. Blood group as well as tissue typing and HLA antibody screen are also checked. Cardiorespiratory investigations include ECG, and chest X-ray. If the patient is younger than 50 years old and has no risk factors these investigations would suffice. If the age of the recipient is greater than 50 years or other cardiac risk factors are present then an exercise ECG should be performed. If this test is positive, or the patient cannot exercise, then a dobutamine stress echo or a myocardial perfusion scan should be performed. All patients with a positive stress test or angina should have coronary angiography. All diabetic patients greater than 40 years old should also undergo coronary angiography as they may have asymptomatic disease. Echocardiography is useful in identifying valvular heart disease as well as regional wall motion abnormalities.[56–58] Some units are more aggressive in their management and have a lower threshold for performing coronary angiography.[59]

5.10 Renal Transplant Procedure

The procedure of renal transplantation has not changed much since the 1950s. It involves implanting the kidney either to the right or left iliac fossa. The approach can be through a pararectal or a modified Rutherford Morison incision. Dissection around the external iliac vein and artery is accomplished before placing vascular clamps and performing the venous anastomosis first, followed by the arterial anastomosis (Figures. 5.7 and 5.8). The ureter is implanted onto the bladder (Figures. 5.9 and 5.10) over a ureteric stent to reduce the risk of a stenosis or a leak developing. This stays in usually for six weeks before it is removed using a cystoscope. The patient usually stays in hospital for five to seven days. After discharge the patient is regularly followed up in a transplant clinic.

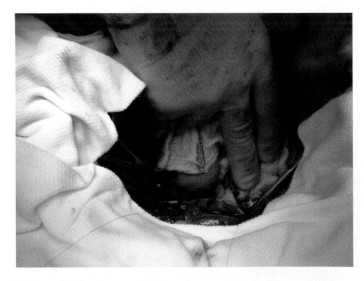

Figure 5.7 Renal vein to external iliac vein anastomosis during a kidney transplant.

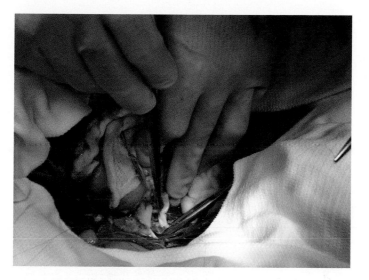

Figure 5.8 Renal artery to external iliac artery anastomosis.

5.11 Complications

5.11.1 Short-term complications

5.11.1.1 *Post-operative bleeding*

This is usually recognised by a reduction in blood pressure associated with an increase in heart rate. Other evidence includes pain and swelling around the wound, a palpable haematoma and a reduction in haemoglobin.[60] There may be excessive blood in the drain but a blocked drain can be misleading. Intravenous fluids and blood products are usually necessary. If the bleeding continues despite these, or if there is pressure from the developing haematoma onto the ureter or renal vessels, exploratory surgery will be required to stop the bleeding and evacuate the haematoma.

5.11.1.2 *Renal artery thrombosis*

Renal artery thrombosis should be suspected if there is a sudden and unexpected reduction in urine output.[60,61] In such cases surgical exploration should be performed as there is little time before the kidney can be saved. This may be related to an intimal tear of the donor renal artery.

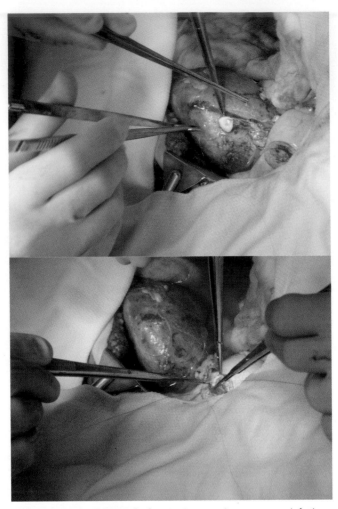

Figures 5.9 (above) and 5.10 (below) A ureteric anastomosis being performed.

5.11.1.3 *Renal vein thrombosis*

Renal vein thrombosis can present with haematuria, pain, and reduction in urine output.[60] Ultrasound scan (USS) may show diastolic reversal of flow in the renal vein as well as loss of flow in the renal vein.[62] Immediate exploration is necessary but in most cases this results in removal of the kidney.

5.11.1.4 *Rejection*

Hyperacute rejection is very rare these days as patients undergo a cross-match prior to proceeding to transplantation, which detects preformed deleterious antibodies that would result in an immunologically incompatible transplant.

Cell-mediated acute rejection is the most common type of rejection and comes in two forms. Tubulointerstitial cell-mediated rejection is characterised by lymphocytic infiltration of the interstitium and the tubules. The interstitium is oedematous. Cell-mediated vascular rejection is characterised by lymphocytic infiltration of the vascular intima. The endothelial cells of the arteries are swollen.[63,64]

Cell-mediated rejection may present with a rise in serum creatinine only. Other signs may include pain over the graft, raised temperature, reduction in urine output, and fluid retention. This is usually treated with intravenous methylprednisolone for three days.[63] Resistant rejection is treated with intravenous ATG for ten days, titrated according to the CD3 count in the recipient's blood.

Antibody-mediated acute rejection is characterised by neutrophilic and lymphocytic infiltration of the arterial wall, endothelial cell damage and thrombosis. Other criteria for antibody-mediated rejection include peritubular capillary staining for C4d as well as the presence of donor-specific antibodies.[65] C4d is a split component of C4 of the classical pathway of complement. Treatment is based on intravenous immunoglobulin (IVIG) and plasmapheresis but newer treatments, like bortezomib (proteasome inhibitor), are currently being evaluated.[63,66]

5.11.1.5 *Urinary obstruction*

Immediate flushing of the urinary catheter should follow any sudden reduction in urine output in the early post-operative period. This will usually solve any problems such as clots in the lumen of the catheter. If there is no improvement in the urinary output, other causes should be investigated. If the urinary catheter has already been removed, urinary retention may be due to an enlarged prostate gland.

A urinary stenosis that becomes obvious after the ureteric stent is removed needs to be treated with a percutaneous nephrostomy and reinsertion of

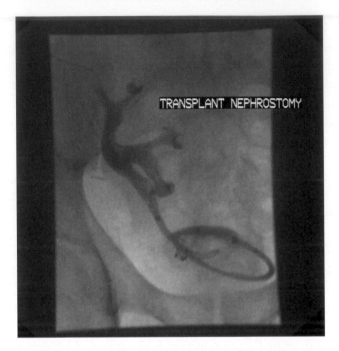

Figure 5.11 Nephrostomy following the diagnosis of ureteric obstruction. This was made following a rise in creatinine after stent removal and detection of hydronephrosis on ultrasound scan.

ureteric stent for three months (Figure 5.11). If this reoccurs or if the ureteric stenosis is long, surgical reimplantation of the ureter is necessary.[67,68]

5.11.1.6 *Haematuria*

This usually resolves within a few days. Bladder clots may require a washout and can cause outflow obstruction.

5.11.1.7 *Urinary leak*

A urinary leak can present with a severe wound pain. A high serum creatinine is due to the urine being reabsorbed and the creatinine not being excreted. Fluid may leak from the wound if the drain has already been removed. A cystogram is useful in detecting a leak near the ureteric anastomosis.

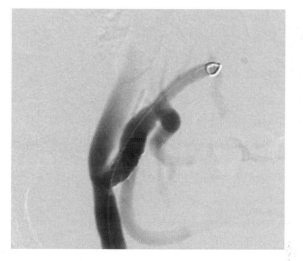

Figure 5.12 Transplant renal artery stenosis treated by percutaneous transluminal angioplasty and stenting.

If the leak is small and the ureteric stent is still *in situ*, conservative management may be employed. Sometimes a percutaneous nephrostomy tube is necessary to divert the urine and allow healing. If the leak is large and it is felt that it will not heal, surgery is required with reimplantation of the ureter.[67,68]

5.11.1.8 *Renal transplant artery stenosis*

Renal transplant artery stenosis is present in 3 to 4% of transplant cases.[69,70] A significant stenosis would show a Doppler velocity of more than 2 m/sec. In addition, the velocity gradient between stenotic and prestenotic areas is more than 2 : 1.[61] The most common treatment is percutaneous transluminal angioplasty and stenting (Figure 5.12) as the results are good and the morbidity is low.[71] Surgical treatment is rarely necessary.

5.11.1.9 *Lymphocele*

This can result from drainage from lymphatics divided at the time of recipient iliac vessel dissection or from the donor kidney. If large, this may cause ureteric obstruction and require drainage and insertion of a sclerosant such as bedadine to obliterate, or surgery to drain into the abdominal cavity.[72,73] The latter can be open or laparoscopic.

5.11.1.10 *Recurrent renal disease*

IgA nephropathy may occur in the new graft in 20 to 60% of cases. Focal Segmental Glomerulosclerosis can occur in up to 30% of cases. Both of these conditions recur in over 80% of patients who proceed to have a second transplant.[74] These issues need to be discussed thoroughly with the potential recipients prior to transplantation.

5.11.2 Long-term complications

The most common cause of death after adult renal transplantation is due to cardiovascular disease, followed by cancer.[76] Post-transplant immunosuppression contributes to these causes in many ways. Cyclosporine is associated with hypertension and hyperlipidaemia. Tacrolimus doubles the risk of diabetes after transplantation.[75] Steroids and sirolimus are associated with hyperlipidaemia but the latter reduces the risk of cancer.[76] Mycophenolate mofetil is also associated with less risk of cancer. On the contrary, azathioprine and calcineurin inhibitors seem to have an increased risk for cancer. The overall incidence of cancer in the transplant population is three to five times that of the general population.[77]

Immunosuppression also increases the risk of infection after transplantation. The risk of cytomegalovirus in high-risk recipients has been reduced with the prophylactic use of valganciclovir.[78] BK is a polyomavirus that has become more prevalent with the use of stronger immunosuppression. Treatment includes reduction of immunosuppression and the use of cidofovir, leflunomide or IVIG.[79] Graft loss is still high in the presence of BK virus.[80]

Furthermore, steroids are associated with reduction in bone mineral density. This is worse in the first few months after transplantation. Patients should have bone densitometry at regular intervals and treated medically as necessary.[81]

Tubular atrophy and interstitial fibrosis are histological signs that give rise to progressive allograft dysfunction. Risk factors for chronic allograft dysfunction include donor age, donor and recipient co-morbidity, delayed graft function, calcineurin inhibitors, acute and subclinical rejection, infection, hypertension and hyperlipidaemia.[82-84] Treatments in an attempt to slow down this process include adequately managing hypertension, hyperlipidemia and infection as well as detection and treatment of subclinical rejection using protocol biopsies and minimisation or elimination of calcineurin inhibitors.[84-86]

5.12 Antibody-Incompatible Transplantation

5.12.1 ABO-incompatible transplantation

Transplantation is limited by the blood group incompatibility between the donor and the recipient. Some 30% of potential renal transplant living donors that come forward are not of the same blood type (ABO-incompatible or ABO-I) to their recipient. The largest experience in ABO-I transplantation comes from Japan where for cultural reasons cadaveric transplantation is constrained. Since 1989, more than 1,000 such cases have been performed in Japan. They account for 18% of all living donor kidney transplants. Since 2001 the one-year and three-year graft survival rates have increased to 96% and 94%, respectively, and are therefore comparable to those of ABO-compatible transplants.[87]

Early approaches in accomplishing ABO-I transplantation included performing a splenectomy at the time of transplantation but more recently this has been substituted by giving rituximab (Roche, Basel, Switzerland). This is a genetically engineered chimaeric murine/human monoclonal antibody directed against the CD20 antigen on B cells. It prevents the formation of new alloantibody-producing plasma cells by eliminating precursor B cells. Rituximab has been used successfully as adjunctive therapy to pre-transplant apheresis protocols, notably in Sweden and Germany but also in the UK, the Netherlands, Switzerland, Greece, France, Spain and Australia.[88-90]

In addition to rituximab, the process of rendering the patient ready for an ABO-incompatible transplant includes pre-transplant plasmapheresis or immunoadsorption to remove IgG and IgM antibodies against the ABO group of the potential recipient to a concentration below a clinically significant titer (typically IgG titer ≤8). Immunoadsorption (GlycoSorb ABO; Glycorex Transplantation AB, Lund, Sweden) has the advantage over plasmapheresis in that it specifically depletes anti-A or anti-B antibodies, only therefore reducing the potential for bleeding due to removal of clotting factors and infectious complications due to the removal of protective antibodies.[88,89] The disadvantage is that this method is more expensive.

The largest study involving rituximab and immunoadsorption comes from Sweden and Germany. This describes a three-centre experience of 60 ABO-incompatible transplants. Two of these grafts were lost after a mean follow-up of 17.5 months (non-compliance and death with a functioning graft). These cases were compared with 274 patients who underwent ABO-compatible kidney transplantation. Graft survival was 97% for the ABO-incompatible compared with 95% for the ABO-compatible. Patient survival was 98% in both groups. There was no late rebound of antibodies and there were no humoral rejections. These results are excellent.[88] The three-year results are similarly very good.[89]

Other approaches include the use of alemtuzumab (Campath, Genzyme Corporation, Cambridge, MA) instead of rituximab with tacrolimus monotherapy after the seventh day. Results are overall very good but antibody-mediated rejection seems to be higher. This is associated with HLA-donor-specific antibodies.[91]

5.13 HLA-Incompatible Transplantation

Patients who have had previous transplants, blood transfusions or pregnancies may become sensitised, that is, develop anti-HLA antibodies. These antibodies would increase the risk of the patient having a positive crossmatch and therefore result in a longer waiting time on the cadaveric waiting list.

There have been two major desensitisation protocols produced over the last few years. The first one involves giving high-dose IVIG and the second one low-dose IVIG and plasmapheresis. High-dose IVIG protocol entails giving monthly infusions (2 gm/kg) of IVIG. Low-dose IVIG protocol involves plasmapheresis and giving low-dose IVIG (100 mg/kg) after each session. Rituximab is sometimes included in these protocols. The results of HLA-incompatible transplantation are similar to those from diseased donor transplantation.[92,93]

Table 5.2 The number of paired exchange kidney donors and altruistic kidney donors in the UK.[98]

Year	Paired exchange donors	Altruistic donors
2007–2008	4	6
2008–2009	16	15

5.14 Pair Exchange and Non-Directed Altruistic Donation

The law surrounding organ donation in the UK is provided by the Human Tissue Act 2004 for England, Wales and Northern Ireland, and the Human Tissue (Scotland) Act 2006. This allows more flexibility in living kidney donation such as pair exchange and non-directed altruistic donation.[94,95]

These methods are also possible in other countries such as the Netherlands and the USA.[92,96]

Table 5.2 shows the number of transplants performed following pair exchange and non-directed altruistic donation in the UK. The numbers are small but still increasing. Most transplants resulting from pair donation so far have been from two-way exchanges. There have been a handful of three-way exchanges. In the USA there has been a chain of paired kidney donations resulting in ten kidney transplants over a period of eight months.[97]

5.15 Immunosuppression

There are a myriad number of immunosuppression protocols based on a relatively small number of established immunosuppressive drugs and depleting antibodies.

5.15.1 Immunosuppressive drugs

5.15.1.1 *Steroids*

Steroids have been used in transplantation since the early 1960s.[99] They inhibit the expression of multiple cytokine genes thus inhibiting T-cell activation at different stages of the process.

5.15.1.2 *Azathioprine*

Azathioprine, is a derivative of 6-mercaptopurine. It has been in use since the early 1960s[99] but its use over the last ten years has diminished. This has been due to the introduction of mycophenolate mofetil.

5.15.1.3 *Cyclosporine*

Cyclosporine is of fungal origin and is a small cyclic polypeptide. This is a calcineurin inhibitor that forms a complex with a cytoplasmic receptor protein called cyclophilin. The complex then binds to calcineurin and inhibits the expression of cytokine genes, like those for IL-2, that normally promote T-cell activation. Thus lymphocyte proliferation is also inhibited.[63]

5.15.1.4 *Tacrolimus*

Tacrolimus, like cyclosporine, is a calcineurin inhibitor that forms a complex with tacrolimus-binding protein. This complex also inhibits lymphocyte proliferation by limiting IL-2 expression.

Tacrolimus is a macrolide antibiotic that is isolated from *Streptomyces tsukubaensis*. Both tacrolimus and cyclosporine require drug monitoring to achieve optimal levels to avoid toxicity or rejection.[63]

5.15.1.5 *Mycophenolate mofetil*

Mycophenolate mofetil (Cellcept) was introduced in the mid 1990s as a replacement for Azathioprine. It is a fermentation product of *Penicillium* species. It is a prodrug and its active compound is mycophenolic acid. This inhibits the enzyme inosine monophosphate dehydrogenase that results in depletion of guanosine nucleotides necessary in lymphocyte proliferation. Myfortic is an enteric coated form of mycophenolic acid and was introduced in 2004. Drug monitoring is not necessary for either of these drugs.[63,100]

5.15.1.6 *Sirolimus*

Sirolimus, also known as rapamycin, is an mTOR (mammalian target of rapamycin) inhibitor that disrupts the process of cell division. It is a macrolide antibiotic and was introduced in 1999. Everolimus (Certican) is also an mTOR inhibitor but has a reduced half-life.[63,101,102]

5.15.2 Depleting antibodies

5.15.2.1 *Thymoglobulin*

This is a polyclonal antibody derived from rabbits that have been immunised with human lymphoid tissue. Thymoglobulin has gained popularity as an induction agent in the USA over the last few years.[103] In the UK, it is usually used for steroid-resistant rejection even though some units use it for higher immunological risk transplants.

5.15.2.2 *Basiliximab*

Basiliximab (Simulect) is an anti–CD25 monoclonal antibody that binds to the IL-2 receptor on T cells. IL-2-mediated responses are therefore blocked. It is used as an induction agent in order to reduce the incidence of rejection soon after surgery. Daclizumab (Zenapax) is a similar antibody but it is no longer in production.[104]

5.15.2.3 *Rituximab*

Rituximab is an anti–CD20 monoclonal antibody that affects B lymphocytes early on in their developmental stage. It results in the depletion of these cells for 6 to 12 months. It is used in ABO-incompatible transplantation as well as HLA-incompatible transplantation.[88,92]

5.15.2.4 *Alemtuzumab*

Alemtuzumab (Campath) is another monoclonal antibody directed against CD52. It is mainly used as an induction agent but can also be used for treating rejection as well as for antibody-incompatible transplantation.[105]

5.16 Conclusions

Renal transplantation is the gold-standard treatment for fit patients with end-stage renal failure. This is because patient survival is better after transplantation when compared to that of patients on dialysis awaiting transplantation[15] and because the quality of life improves after transplantation.[16] The latter includes general quality of life, as well as physical and psychosocial functioning.

Over the last few years there has been a drive toward achieving pre-emptive transplantation, as this is associated with less graft failure and mortality compared to patients having a transplant after commencing dialysis.[106]

Over the last ten years there has been an increase in the number of live donor transplants. This has been achieved with the introduction of minimally invasive live donor procedures as well as the introduction of antibody-incompatible transplantation, pair exchange and non-directed altruistic transplantation. Over the next few years we will observe the introduction of a number of new immunosuppressive drugs, which hopefully will improve the outcomes even further.[107]

References

1. Hamilton, D.N.H. and Reid, W.A. (1984). Yu Yu Voronoy and the First Human Kidney Allograft, *Surg Gynecol Obstet*, **159**, 289–294.
2. Merrill, J.P. *et al.* (1956). Successful Homotransplantation of the Human Kidney Between Identical Twins, *JAMA*, **160**, 277–282.
3. Merrill, J.P. *et al.* (1956). Renal Homotransplantation in Identical Twins, *Surg Forum*, **6**, 432–436.
4. Calne, R. (1999). *The Ultimate Gift: The Story of Britain's Premier Transplant Surgeon*, Headline Book Publishing, London.
5. Starzl, T.E. (1992). *The Puzzle People*, University of Pittsburgh Press, Pittsburgh.
6. Calne, R.Y. *et al.* (1966). Further Observations on Renal Transplants in Man from Cadaveric Donors, *Br Med J*, **2(5526)**, 1345–1351.
7. Diethelm, A.G. *et al.* (1974). Clinical Evaluation of Equine Antithymocyte Globulin in Recipients of Renal Allografts: Analysis of Survival, Renal Function, Rejection, Histocompatibility, and Complications, *Ann Surg*, **180(1)**, 20–28.
8. Calne, R. (2004). Cyclosporine as a Milestone in Immunosuppression, *Transplant Proc*, **36(2 Suppl)**, 13S–15S.
9. Calne, R. *et al.* (1981). Cyclosporin A in Cadaveric Organ Transplantation, *Br Med J*, **282**, 934–936.
10. Starzl, T.E. *et al.* (1989). FK 506 for Liver, Kidney, and Pancreas Transplantation, *Lancet*, **2(8670)**, 1000–1004.
11. Webster, A.C. *et al.* (2005). Tacrolimus versus Cyclosporin as Primary Immunosuppression for Kidney Transplant Recipients: Meta-analysis and Meta-regression of Randomised Trial Data, *BMJ*, **331(7520)**, 810.

12. Webster, A.C. *et al.* (2005). Tacrolimus versus Cyclosporin as Primary Immunosuppression for Kidney Transplant Recipients, *Cochrane Database Syst Rev*, **(4)**, CD003961.

13. Gralla, J. and Wiseman, A.C. (2010). The Impact of IL2ra Induction Therapy in Kidney Transplantation Using Tacrolimus- and Mycophenolate-Based Immunosuppression, *Transplantation*, **90(6)**, 639–644.

14. Fuggle, S.V. *et al.* (2010). Factors Affecting Graft and Patient Survival After Live Donor Kidney Transplantation in the UK, *Transplantation*, **89(6)**, 694–701.

15. Johnson, R.J. *et al.* (2010). Factors Influencing Outcome After Deceased Heart-Beating Donor Kidney Transplantation in the United Kingdom: An Evidence Base for a New National Kidney Allocation Policy, *Transplantation*, **89(4)**, 379–386.

16. Wolfe, R.A. *et al.* (1999). Comparison of Mortality in all Patients on Dialysis, Patients on Dialysis Awaiting Transplantation, and Recipients of a First Cadaveric Transplant, *N Engl J Med*, **341(23)**, 1725–1730.

17. Landreneau, K., Lee, K. and Landreneau, M.D. (2010). Quality of Life in Patients Undergoing Hemodialysis and Renal Transplantation: A Meta analytic Review, *Nephrol Nurs J*, **37(1)**, 37–44.

18. Hariharan, S. *et al.* (2000). Improved Graft Survival After Renal Transplantation in the United States, 1988 to 1996, *N Engl J Med*, **342(9)**, 605–612.

19. Domínguez-Gil, B. and Pascual, J. (2008). Living Donor Renal Transplant in Spain: A Great Opportunity, *Nefrologia*, **28(2)**, 143–147.

20. Axelrod, D.A. *et al.* (2010). Kidney and Pancreas Transplantation in the United States, 1999–2008: The Changing Face of Living Donation, *Am J Transplant*, **10(2)**, 987–1002.

21. Horvat, L.D., Shariff, S.Z. and Garg, A.X. (2009). Donor Nephrectomy Outcomes: Global Trends in the Rates of Living Kidney Donation, *Kidney Int*, **75**, 1088–1098.

22. NHSBT. (2010). *Annual Review 2009–2010*. Available at: http://www.nhsbt. nhs.uk/annualreview/index.asp (accessed 29 October 2010).

23. NHSBT (no date). *UK Activity Report 2008–2009*. Available at: http://www.uktransplant.org.uk/ukt/statistics/transplant_activity_report/archive_activity_reports/archive_activity_reports.jsp (accessed 28 October 2010).

24. BTS. (2011). *Active BTS Standards and Guidelines*. Available at: http://www.bts.org.uk/transplantation/standards-and-guidelines/ (accessed 24 October 2010).

25. Kessaris, N. *et al.* (2010). *Live Donor Kidney Transplantation. Living Related Transplantation*, World Scientific, Singapore.

26. Hakim, N. *et al.* (2010). A Fast and Safe Living Donor 'Finger-Assisted' Nephrectomy Technique: Results of 359 Cases, *Transplant Proc*, **42**, 165–170.

27. Ratner, L.E. *et al.* (1995). Laparoscopic Live Donor Nephrectomy. *Transplantation*, **60**, 1047–1049.

28. Chandak, P. *et al.* (2009). How Safe is Hand-Assisted Laparoscopic Donor Nephrectomy? Results of 200 Live Donor Nephrectomies by Two Different Techniques, *Nephrol Dial Transplant*, **24(1)**, 293–297.

29. Gjertsen, H. *et al.* (2006). Introduction of Hand-Assisted Retroperitoneoscopic Living Donor Nephrectomy at Karolinska University Hospital Huddinge, *Transplant Proc*, **38(8)**, 2644–2645.

30. Fronek, J.P., Chang, R.W. and Morsy, M.A. (2006). Hand-Assisted Retroperitoneoscopic Living Donor Nephrectomy: First UK Experience, *Nephrol Dial Transplant*, **21(9)**, 2674–2675.

31. Canes, D. *et al.* (2010). Laparo-Endoscopic Single Site (LESS) versus Standard Laparoscopic Left Donor Nephrectomy: Matched-Pair Comparison, *Eur Urol*, **57(1)**, 95–101.

32. Allaf, M.E. *et al.* (2010). Laparoscopic Live Donor Nephrectomy with Vaginal Extraction: Initial Report, *Am J Transplant*, **10(6)**, 1473–1477.

33. Alcaraz, A. *et al.* (2010). Transvaginal Notes-Assisted Laparoscopic Living Donor Nephrectomy, *Am J Transplant*, **10(S4)**, 105.

34. Jacobs, S.C. *et al.* (2004). Laparoscopic Donor Nephrectomy: The University of Maryland 6-Year Experience, *J Urol*, **171(1)**, 47–51.

35. Cooper, M. *et al.* (2006). Laparoscopic Donor Nephrectomy for Transplantation: 10 Years and 1000 Consecutive Cases, *Am J Transplant*, **6(S2)**, 286.

36. Melcher, M.L. *et al.* (2005). More than 500 Consecutive Laparoscopic Donor Nephrectomies Without Conversion or Repeated Surgery, *Arch Surg*, **140**, 835–839.

37. Matas, A.J. *et al.* (2003). Morbidity and Mortality After Living Kidney Donation, 1999–2001: Survey of United States Transplant Centers, *Am J Transplant*, **3(7)**, 830–834.

38. Segev, D.L. *et al.* (2010). Perioperative Mortality and Long-Term Survival Following Live Kidney Donation, *JAMA*, **303(10)**, 959–966.

39. Hadjianastassiou, V.G. *et al.* (2007). 2509 Living Donor Nephrectomies, Morbidity and Mortality, Including the UK Introduction of Laparoscopic Donor Surgery, *Am J Transplant*, **7(11)**, 2532–2537.

40. Oyen, O. *et al.* (2005). Laparoscopic versus Open Living-Donor Nephrectomy: Experiences from a Prospective, Randomized, Single-center Study Focusing on Donor Safety, *Transplantation*, **79**, 1236–1240.

41. Wolf, J.S. *et al.* (2001). Randomized Controlled Trial of Hand-Assisted Laparoscopic versus Open Surgical Live Donor Nephrectomy, *Transplantation*, **72**, 284–290.

42. Simforoosh, N. *et al.* (2005). Comparison of Laparoscopic and Open Donor Nephrectomy: A Randomized Controlled Trial, *BJU Int*, **95**, 851–855.

43. Lewis, G.R. *et al.* (2004). A Comparison of Traditional Open, Minimal-Incision Donor Nephrectomy and Laparoscopic Donor Nephrectomy, *Transpl Int*, **17**, 589–595.

44. Kokkinos, C. *et al.* (2007). Comparison of Laparoscopic versus Hand-Assisted Live Donor Nephrectomy, *Transplantation*, **83**, 41–47.

45. Friedman, A.L. *et al.* (2006). Fatal and Nonfatal Hemorrhagic Complications of Living Kidney Donation, *Ann Surg*, **243**, 126–130.

46. Boudville, N., Prasad, G.V. and Knoll, G. (2006). Meta-analysis: Risk for Hypertension in Living Kidney Donors, *Ann Intern Med*, **145**, 185–196.

47. Ibrahim, H.N. *et al.* (2009). Long-Term Consequences of Kidney Donation, *N Engl J Med*, **360(5)**, 459–469.

48. Organ Donation. 2010. *Monthly Statistics*. Available at: http://www.organdonation.nhs.uk/ukt/statistics/latest_statistics/monthly.jsp (accessed 18 September 2010).

49. Organ Procurement and Transplantation Network (OPTN) Data, US Department of Health and Human Services. Available at: http://optn.transplant.hrsa.gov/latestData/rptData.asp (accessed 18 September 2010).

50. Kootstra, G., Daemen, J.H.C. and Oomen, A.P.A. (1995). Categories of Non-Heart-Beating Donors, *Transplant Proc*, **27**, 2893–2894.

51. Chaib, E. (2008). Non Heart-Beating Donors in England, *Clinics*, **63(1)**, 121–134.

52. Barlow, A.D. *et al.* (2009). Case-Matched Comparison of Long-Term Results of Non-Heart-Beating and Heart-Beating Donor Renal Transplants, *Br J Surg*, **96(6)**, 685–691.

53. Moustafellos, P. *et al.* (2007). The Influence of Pulsatile Preservation in Kidney Transplantation From Non-Heart-Beating Donors, *Transplant Proc*, **39(5)**, 1323–1325.

54. Moers, C. *et al.* (2009). Machine Perfusion or Cold Storage in Deceased-Donor Kidney Transplantation, *N Engl J Med*, **360(1)**, 7–19.

55. Watson, C.J. *et al.* (2010). Cold Machine Perfusion versus Static Cold Storage of Kidneys Donated After Cardiac Death: A UK Multicenter Randomized Controlled Trial, *Am J Transplant*, **10(9)**, 1991–1999.

56. Summers, D.M. *et al.* (2010). Analysis of Factors that Affect Outcome After Transplantation of Kidneys Donated After Cardiac Death in the UK: A Cohort Study, *Lancet*, Oct 16, **376(9749)**,1303–1311.

57. Torpey, N. *et al.* (2010). *Renal Transplantation*, Oxford University Press, Oxford.

58. Pilmore, H.L. (2009). Review Article. Coronary Artery Stenoses: Detection and Revascularization in Renal Disease, *Nephrology*, **14(6)**, 537–543.

59. Kumar, N. *et al.* (2010). Is Pre-Emptive Coronary Artery Revascularisation Responsible for a Low Number of Cardiac Events Following Transplantation in the Short and Medium Term? *Am J Transplant*, **10(S4)**, 241.

60. Morris, P.J. and Knechtle, S.J. (2008). *Kidney Transplantation: Principles and Practice*, Sixth Edition, Saunders, Elsevier, Philadelphia.

61. Akbar, S.A. *et al.* (2005). Complications of Renal Transplantation, *Radiographics*, **25(5)**, 1335–1356.

62. Schwenger, V. *et al.* (2006). Color Doppler Ultrasonography in the Diagnostic Evaluation of Renal Allografts, *Nephron Clin Pract*, **104(3)**, c107–c112.

63. Danovitch, G.M. (2010). *Handbook of Kidney Transplantation*, Fifth Edition, Lippincott Williams & Wilkins, Wolters Kluwer, Philadelphia.

64. Halloran, P.F. (2010). T Cell-Mediated Rejection of Kidney Transplants: A Personal Viewpoint, *Am J Transplant*, **10(5)**, 1126–1134.

65. Truong, L.D. *et al.* (2007). Acute Antibody-Mediated Rejection of Renal Transplant: Pathogenetic and Diagnostic Considerations, *Arch Pathol Lab Med*, **131(8)**, 1200–1208.

66. Everly, J.J. *et al.* (2009). Proteasome Inhibition for Antibody-Mediated Rejection, *Curr Opin Organ Transplant*, **14(6)**, 662–666.

67. Al-Shaer, M.B. and Al-Midani, A. (2005). The Management of Urological Complications in Renal Transplant Patients, *Saudi J Kidney Dis Transpl*, **16(2)**, 176–180.

68. Zavos, G. *et al.* (2008). Urological Complications: Analysis and Management of 1525 Consecutive Renal Transplantations, *Transplant Proc*, **40(5)**, 1386–1390.

69. Patel, N.H. *et al.* (2001). Renal Arterial Stenosis in Renal Allografts: Retrospective Study of Predisposing Factors and Outcome After Percutaneous Transluminal Angioplasty, *Radiology*, **219(3)**, 663–667.

70. Patel, U. (2003). Doppler Ultrasound for Detection of Renal Transplant Artery Stenosis-Threshold Peak Systolic Velocity Needs to be Higher in a Low-Risk or Surveillance Population, *Clin Radiol*, **58(10)**, 772–777.

71. Ridgway, D. *et al.* (2006). Primary Endoluminal Stenting of Transplant Renal Artery Stenosis from Cadaver and Non-Heart-Beating Donor Kidneys, *Clin Transplant*, **20(3)**, 394–400.

72. Zomorrodi, A. and Buhluli, A. (2007). Instillation of Povidone Iodine to Treat Lymphocele and Leak of Lymph After Renal Transplantation, *Saudi J Kidney Dis Transpl*, **18(4)**, 621–624.

73. Iwan-Zietek, I. *et al.* (2009). Minimally Invasive Methods for the Treatment of Lymphocele After Kidney Transplantation, *Transplant Proc*, **41(8)**, 3073–3076.

74. Golgert, W.A., Appel, G.B. and Hariharan, S. (2008). Recurrent Glomerulonephritis After Renal Transplantation: An Unsolved Problem, *Clin J Am Soc Nephrol*, **3(3)**, 800–807.

75. Webster, A.C. *et al.* (2005). Tacrolimus versus Ciclosporin as Primary Immunosuppression for Kidney Transplant Recipients: Meta-analysis and Meta-regression of Randomised Trial Data, *BMJ*, **331(7520)**, 810.

76. Marcén, R. (2009). Immunosuppressive Drugs in Kidney Transplantation: Impact on Patient Survival, and Incidence of Cardiovascular Disease, Malignancy and Infection, *Drugs*, **69(16)**, 2227–2243.

77. Wong, G. and Chapman, J.R. (2008). Cancers After Renal Transplantation, *Transplant Rev (Orlando)*, **22(2)**, 141–149.

78. Humar, A. *et al.* (2010). The Efficacy and Safety of 200 Days Valganciclovir Cytomegalovirus Prophylaxis in High-Risk Kidney Transplant Recipients, *Am J Transplant*, **10(5)**, 1228–1237.

79. Johnston, O. *et al.* (2010). Treatment of Polyomavirus Infection in Kidney Transplant Recipients: A Systematic Review, *Transplantation*, **89(9)**, 1057–1070.

80. Montagner, J. *et al.* (2010). BKV-Infection in Kidney Graft Dysfunction, *Braz J Infect Dis*, **14(2)**, 170–174.

81. Matuszkiewicz-Rowińska, J. (2010). KDIGO Clinical Practice Guidelines for the Diagnosis, Evaluation, Prevention, and Treatment of Mineral and Bone Disorders in Chronic Kidney Disease, *Pol Arch Med Wewn*, **120(7–8)**, 300–306.

82. Li, C. and Yang, C.W. (2009). The Pathogenesis and Treatment of Chronic Allograft Nephropathy, *Nat Rev Nephrol*, **5(9)**, 513–519.

83. Yates, P.J. and Nicholson, M.L. (2006). The Aetiology and Pathogenesis of Chronic Allograft Nephropathy, *Transpl Immunol*, **16(3–4)**, 148–157.

84. Nankivell, B.J. and Chapman, J.R. (2006). Chronic Allograft Nephropathy: Current Concepts and Future Directions, *Transplantation*, **81(5)**, 643–654.

85. Campistol, J.M. *et al.* (2009). Chronic Allograft Nephropathy — A Clinical Syndrome: Early Detection and the Potential Role of Proliferation Signal Inhibitors, *Clin Transplant*, **23(6)**, 769–777.

86. Wali, R.K. and Weir, M.R. (2008). Chronic Allograft Dysfunction: Can We Use Mammalian Target of Rapamycin Inhibitors to Replace Calcineurin Inhibitors to Preserve Graft Function? *Curr Opin Organ Transplant*, **13(6)**, 614–621.

87. Sonoda, T. *et al.* (2003). Outcome of 3 Years of Immunosuppression with Tacrolimus in More than 1,000 Renal Transplant Recipients in Japan, *Transplantation*, **75(2)**, 199–204.

88. Tyden, G. *et al.* (2007). Implementation of a Protocol for ABO-Incompatible Kidney Transplantation: A Three-Center Experience with 60 Consecutive Transplantations, *Transplantation*, **83**, 1153–1155.

89. Genberg, H. *et al.* (2008). ABO-Incompatible Kidney Transplantation Using Antigen-Specific Immunoadsorption and Rituximab: a 3-Year Follow-up, *Transplantation*, **85(12)**, 1745–1754.

90. Tydén, G. (2006). Cost-Effectiveness of ABO-Incompatible Kidney Transplantations, *Transplantation*, **82(2)**, 166–167.

91. Galliford, J. *et al.* (2010). Antibody-Mediated Rejection After ABO Incompatible Living Donor Renal Transplantation is Mainly Associated with HLA Donor Specific Antibodies, *Am J Transplant*, **10(S4)**, 164.

92. Montgomery, R.A. (2010). Renal Transplantation Across HLA and ABO Antibody Barriers: Integrating Paired Donation into Desensitization Protocols, *Am J Transplant*, **10(3)**, 449–457.

93. Jordan, S.C., Peng, A. and Vo, A.A. (2009). Therapeutic Strategies in Management of the Highly HLA-Sensitized and ABO-Incompatible Transplant Recipients, *Contrib Nephrol*, **162**, 13–26.

94. HTA. (2004). *Human Tissue Act 2004*. Available at: http://www.hta. gov.uk/legislationpoliciesandcodesofpractice/legislation/humantissueact.cfm (accessed 18 September 2010).

95. Mahendran, A.O. and Veitch, P.S. (2007). Paired Exchange Programmes Can Expand the Live Kidney Donor Pool, *BJS*, **94**, 657–664.

96. de Klerk, M. *et al.* (2005). The Dutch National Living Donor Kidney Exchange Program, *Am J Transplant*, **5(9)**, 2302–2305.

97. Rees, M.A. *et al.* (2009). A Nonsimultaneous, Extended, Altruistic-Donor Chain, *N Engl J Med*, **360(11)**, 1096–1101.

98. Organ Donation. (No date). *Archive Activity Reports*. Available at: http://www. organdonation.nhs.uk/ukt/statistics/transplant_activity_report / archive_acti vity_ reports/archive_ activity_reports.jsp (accessed 02 November 2010).

99. Woodruff, M. (1969). Immunosuppression and its Complications, *Proc R Soc Med*, April, **62(4)**, 411–416.

100. Villarroel, M.C., Hidalgo, M. and Jimeno, A. (2009). Mycophenolate Mofetil: An Update, *Drugs Today (Barc)*, **45(7)**, 521–532.

101. Marcén, R. (2009). Immunosuppressive Drugs in Kidney Transplantation: Impact on Patient Survival, and Incidence of Cardiovascular Disease, Malignancy and Infection, *Drugs*, **69(16)**, 2227–2243.

102. Rostaing, L. and Kamar, N. (2010). mTOR Inhibitor/Proliferation Signal Inhibitors: Entering or Leaving the Field? *J Nephrol*, **23(2)**, 133–142.

103. Brennan, D.C. *et al.* (2006). Rabbit Antithymocyte Globulin versus Basiliximab in Renal Transplantation, *N Engl J Med*, **355(19)**, 1967–1977.

104. Webster, A.C. *et al.* (2010). Interleukin 2 Receptor Antagonists for Kidney Transplant Recipients, *Cochrane Database Syst Rev*, **(1)**, CD003897.

105. Pham, P.T. *et al.* (2009). The Evolving Role of Alemtuzumab (Campath-1H) in Renal Transplantation, *Drug Des Devel Ther*, **3**, 41–49.

106. Kasiske, B.L. *et al.* (2002). Preemptive Kidney Transplantation: The Advantage and the Advantaged, *J Am Soc Nephrol*, **13**, 1358–1364.

107. Cooper, J.E. and Wiseman, A.C. (2010). Novel Immunosuppressive Agents in Kidney Transplantation, *Clin Nephrol*, **73(5)**, 333–343.

6

Pancreas Transplantation

Asim Syed and Nadey S. Hakim

Diabetes mellitus is associated with a significant morbidity and mortality even in patients with tight glycaemic control.[1,2] With modern developments in pancreas transplantation techniques, better immunosuppression and post operative care bringing about improvements in post-operative complications, patient morbidity and mortality and graft survival, pancreas transplantation has become a curative option for those with diabetes. The price of this cure is a major operation and long-term immunosuppression.

6.1 Indications for Pancreas Transplantation

Pancreas transplantation is indicated in patients diagnosed with diabetes mellitus (DM). The significance of diabetes is such that suffering from diabetes alone is enough to justify accepting the risks of pancreas transplantation. The Diabetes Control and Complications trial not only highlighted the importance of tight glycaemic control, but showed that even patients with a tight glycaemic control had a 5 to 15% risk of developing secondary complications, such as nephropathy, retinopathy and autonomic neuropa-

111

thy.[1−3] The majority of pancreas transplants have been done in patients with an absolute insulin deficiency (Type 1 DM), but more recently they have also been carried out in patients who have become dependent on insulin despite some endogenous insulin production (Type 2 DM).[3]

The key to the appropriate selection of patients to undergo pancreas transplantation lies in a comprehensive multidisciplinary pre-transplant evaluation. Key components of the evaluation include anaesthetic and cardiovascular assessments and management of patient expectations. It is essential for the patient to understand the potential risks and benefits of pancreas transplantation. Exclusion criteria include: active infection or malignancy, current major psychiatric illness or instability, substance abuse, insufficient cardiovascular reserve, and a BMI greater than 25.[4]

Pancreas transplantation can be split into three main categories: simultaneous pancreas-kidney transplantation (SPK), pancreas-after-kidney transplant (PAK) and pancreas transplant alone (PTA).

SPK is the most common transplant procedure and has the greatest one-year and long-term pancreas graft survival rates of all pancreas transplant operations. It also has a better outcome (in terms of one-year graft and patient survival rates) in these patients than kidney transplantation alone.[5] Mostly, both organs come from the same cadaveric donor, but sometimes a cadaveric pancreas is transplanted at the same time as a kidney from a living kidney donor. Rarely are living donor SPKs performed.[2,5]

Solitary pancreas transplants are performed either in diabetic patients without end-stage renal disease (ESRD) (PTA) or in patients who have already had a kidney transplant (PAK).[2,3]

6.2 Procurement and Preservation of the Pancreas

The majority of organs for pancreas transplantation come from cadaveric heart-beating donors (around 95%).[6] The rest are from cadaveric non-heart-beating donors and rarely from living donors (whose procurement is slightly different and not going to be discussed in this chapter).

There are two main techniques of procurement: *in vivo* dissection and en bloc procurement.[7] There is some evidence to suggest that successful *in vivo* dissection is more dependent upon the experience and ability of the operating surgeon.[3,7] En bloc dissection of the liver and pancreas has been shown to have certain advantages, such as reduced warm ischaemic time and better identification of the arterial anatomy, especially aberrant arterial anatomy (in particular aberrant left and right hepatic arteries).[7,8]

The important features required for successful retrieval are the same regardless of technique — minimal handling and shorter dissection time — as donor instability and pancreatic manipulation are well-recognized risk factors for primary graft non-function and graft pancreatitis.[8,9] Most retrieval teams adopt an *in situ* flushing technique that allows flushing and cooling of the intra-abdominal organs with a hypothermic preservation solution (University of Wisconsin solution is still the preferred solution) prior to procurement.[10] The supra coeliac abdominal aorta is clamped and distal aorta is cannulated and flushed with 2–3 litres of the hypothermic preservation solution (a cannula is often placed in the IVC to vent the perfusate).[3,9] This technique must be adopted for procurement from non-heart-beating donors and unstable donors.[7] Some transplant surgeons like perfusion of the portal system as well, to promote rapid cooling of the liver. If this is the case then the portal vein cannula must be placed in the portal vein between the pancreas and the liver in order to dual perfuse the liver and avoid the high perfusion pressures that can occur in the pancreas associated with dual perfusion. Dual perfusion of the pancreas is associated with higher levels of serum amylase and lipase and lower levels of urinary bicarbonate, pH and amylase in the recipients post-transplant, than in those recipients where portal perfusion of the pancreas was not used.[8,9]

6.3 Blood Supply

The pancreas graft is a low microcirculatory organ, has significant intra-pancreatic arterial collateral circulation, and its main blood supply is from the splenic artery and superior mesenteric artery.[10] These need to be vascularly reconstructed before transplantation and are usually anastamosed end to end with a y-graft from the iliac arteries (external and internal to pancreatic arteries and common to recipient) or from the carotids or braciocephalic trunk (there are other methods of reconstructing the arterial supply but these are associated with poorer outcomes).[6,10]

6.4 Preservation Solution

The ideal preservation solution opposes the changes that occur to the organ due to ischaemic damage and during cold storage. Therefore components that are essential to have are: osmotically active substances to suppress cell swelling; an ionic concentration to oppose sodium influx and to help stabilize the cell membrane; buffers to help maintain a steady pH; metabolites for regenerating energy production; inhibitors of the breakdown of important structural proteins, scavengers of oxygen radicals and substances that prevent their formation; and vasoactive substances to increase blood flow during reperfusion.[11]

Hypothermia is associated with osmotic changes causing cellular swelling, and to minimize this most preservation solutions contain uncharged saccharides (mannitol, raffinose, glucose, sucrose) or impermeable anions (gluconate, glycerophosphate, lactobionate) at about 110 to 140 mmol (similar to the concentration of intracellular anions).[11] Tri- and di-saccharides are associated with a better outcome in pancreas preservation and have a direct cytoprotective effect as they help maintain cellular ATP content. Addition of adenine and ribose or adenosine can further help maintain cellular ATP content.[11]

Of the four most common preservation solutions (University of Wisconsin (UW), histidine-tryptophan-keto-glutarate (HTK), Institut-George-Lopes (IGL-1) and Celsior solutions), UW is still the preservation solution of choice for most centres. [11,12] Recently there has been an increase in use of HTK solution for both liver and kidney transplantation.[12] However, in pancreas transplantation it has been shown to be independently associated with an increased risk of graft loss (especially in cold ischaemic times greater than 12 hours) and an increased risk of early graft loss.[12]

6.5 Recipient Operation

Pancreas transplantation can be performed through a midline abdominal incision, J-shaped iliac incision and transverse abdominal incision.[13] The pancreas can then be placed intra- or extra-peritoneally with the organ getting its blood supply from the external iliac or common iliac arteries. The two main areas of controversy are related to the venous drainage and drainage of the exocrine secretions of the pancreas.[6]

The portal vein of the pancreas graft is commonly anastamosed to the iliac vein (external or common) of the recipient. However, recently there has been some debate about this technique as it results in insulin secretion into the systemic circulation, resulting in hyperinsulinaemia, despite normal blood glucose levels.[6,14] Hyperinsulinaemia is known to be associated with accelerated atherosclerotic disease, hypertension and hypercholesterolaemia in non-transplant patients, and there is some concern about this occurring in pancreas-transplant patients with the systemic venous drainage technique.[6,14] An alternative technique, to avoid this, is to anastamose the portal vein from the donor pancreas to the superior mesenteric vein of the recipient. Although there is evidence to suggest that it has comparable short-term graft survival and technical complication rates, there is no evidence to show any metabolic advantages of this technique. Also in the setting of transplantation (especially with the use of steroids and calcinuerin inhibitors) there is no evidence to suggest hyperinsulinaemia has the same effect as in the non-transplant patient. Therefore, the technically simpler systemic venous anastomosis is the preferred choice of most centres.[10]

There are two main options for drainage of the exocrine pancreatic secretions: bladder drainage or enteric drainage.[14] The main advantage of bladder drainage is thought to be the ability to monitor for early rejection by monitoring the urinary amylase level.[6,14] Other advantages are: not contaminating the operating field with enteric contents, and protection of the anastomosis with a Foley catheter.[14] The main *dis*advantage is loss of large amounts of bicarbonate through pancreatic exocrine secretions in the urine, often resulting in a metabolic acidosis.[6] Other disadvantages include recurrent UTIs, chemical cystitis and urethritis, bladder stones, ulceration of the bladder or duodenum leading to haematuria, reflux pancreatitis, dysuria, perineal excoriation and inflammation, ureteral disruption, and strictures.[3,6,10] These complications are thought to be responsible for the resurgence of enteric drainage. According to the International Pancreas Transplant Registry (IPTR), more than 90% of pancreas transplants worldwide were bladder-drained in 1995. However, by 2003, 80%

of pancreas transplants reported to the IPTR, were reported as enterically drained.[3,6,10]

6.6 Immunosuppression

Immunosuppression for pancreas transplantation is very similar to that for kidney transplantation and other solid organs.[3] Immunosuppression therapy can be classified into two main categories: induction and maintenance. There are a variety of different immunosuppressive medications and regimes used by different institutions for both induction and maintenance. However, despite their differences, these medications and regimes all try to achieve the same goals: to prevent acute and chronic rejection with minimal toxicity and minimal increased risk of infection and malignancy, and to maximize organ survival. These goals are the same as those of immunosuppression therapy for any other solid organ transplantation.[3]

Induction immunotherapy usually consists of a short course of an intravenous agent or agents usually targeted at human lymphoid cells, resulting in a significant reduction of these cells, almost to the level that they are undetectable, to help prevent early acute rejection. Antilymphocyte antibody induction therapeutic agents are commonly used.[15]

Maintenance immunotherapy is extremely varied with no clear optimal regime or agent(s).[16] However, tacrolimus/mycophenolate mofetil or tacrolimus/sirolimus with steroid withdrawal, are common mainstay regimens, in modern pancreas transplantation.[15,17,18]

6.7 Outcomes

According to the IPTR, over 30,000 pancreas transplants have been performed worldwide from 16 December 1966 to 31 December 2008.[19] According to the United Network for Organ Sharing (UNOS), the majority of patients undergoing pancreas transplantation, from 2004 to 2008, had an SPK (73%). The remaining pancreas transplants were either transplanted as PAKs (18%) or PTAs (9%), or as part of a multiorgan transplant (or any organ other than kidney) (2%).[19,20] Of those patients that had a PAK, the majority had a live-kidney donor (76%).[19]

Currently, it has yet to be determined whether pancreas transplantation results in increased survival. Gruessner *et al.* published 15-year actuarial patient survival as 56% for SPK, 42% for PAK and 59% for PTA (with pancreas graft survival as 36%, 18% and 16%, respectively), with death of the recipient and chronic rejection being the greatest causes of graft loss at ten years (53% and 33%, respectively).[6] However, there have been several studies that have found comparable survival rates of patients who underwent SPK as those who had a kidney transplant alone (KTA) if the kidney was from a living donor (LD). The survival rate was significantly better than if the kidney was from a deceased donor (DD), with SPK recipients living ten years longer than DD KTA recipients (23.4 years versus 13.9 years).[6,21] The ten-year kidney survival rate was 67% for SPK recipients, 65% for LD KTA recipients and 47% for DD KTA recipients (all of whom had Type 1 DM).[6] SPK recipients also had better renal graft function than the DD KTA recipients at this time.[6] Sollinger *et al.* published SPK recipient survival at 1, 10 and 20 years as 97%, 80% and 58%; kidney survival as 91%, 63% and 38%; and pancreas survival as 88%, 63% and 36%, respectively.[22] Table 6.1 shows patient and graft survival data for diabetic recipients undergoing pancreas and kidney transplants in the US (one-, three- and five-year data from transplants performed in 2003, and ten-year data taken from transplants performed in 1998).[23]

Table 6.1 Patient and graft survival data for diabetic recipients undergoing pancreas and kidney transplants in the US.

		1 year	3 years	5 years	10 years
Pancreas survival (%)	SPK	85.3	79.6	73.6	53.5
	PAK	77.4	61.9	48.7	33.1
	PTA	67.5	46.1	42.9	35
Kidney survival (%)	SPK	92	84.7	77.3	58.8
	LD KTA	96.6	—	77.3	47.8
	DD KTA	89.8	—	64.8	32.3
Patient survival (%)	SPK	95.5	91.7	87.5	71.4
	PAK	95.4	89.8	83.8	65.6
	PTA	93.8	90.7	87.5	75.9
	LD KTA	98.5	—	86.1	61.6
	DD KTA	94.7	—	76.4	45.4

The mortality hazard is lower for SPK recipients than those waiting for a transplant (even at one year).[6,24] Of those patients, 50% on the SPK waiting list die at four years.[6] But it must be remembered that pancreas transplantation is associated with a reduction in survival rate in the first few months (1.5, 2.27 and 2.89 fold reductions at 90 days, for SPK, PTA and PAK recipients, respectively).[6] Pancreas transplant recipients are often very difficult to manage with frequent complications leading to high costs.[21]

6.8 Effects of Pancreas Transplantation on Secondary Complications of Diabetes and Quality of Life

Retinopathy is stabilized and pancreas transplantation has beneficial effects regarding macular oedema. After three years, it may even reduce deterioration in those with advanced eye disease.[6]

Neuropathy improves (motor and sensory after as little as one year, autonomic after five years) continuously in the post–transplant period, as long as the patient is maintained in a normoglycaemic state.[3,14,25]

Atherosclerotic cardiovascular disease has been shown to regress in up to 40% of patients post-pancreas transplantation.[6] There is also evidence to suggest stabilization and even improvement in cardiac autonomic dysfunction, return to normal of diastolic dysfunction, and improvement in cardiac geometry.[6] Patients with a functioning pancreas graft also have a lower incidence of myocardial infarction and pulmonary oedema.[6]

Pancreas transplant within the first few years after a kidney transplant have been shown to halt progression of diabetic glomerulopathy lesions and even start to reverse these lesions after 10 years.[3,6,14,25]

6.9 Quality of Life (QoL)

Quality of life studies report an improvement post transplantation particularly with freedom from dietary restrictions, insulin and blood sugar monitoring.[6,14,25] Also improvements in cognitive function, overall health, pain, physical function and employment opportunities have also been reported.[3,26]

6.10 Surgical Complications of Pancreas Transplantation

Pancreas transplantation is associated with the highest surgical complication rates of all solid organ transplantations.[10,20,27,28] The majority of pancreas grafts lost are due to surgical complications in the early post-transplantation period.[20,27,28] Graft thrombosis is thought to account for almost half of these.[2] Vascular thrombosis is still reported to be the most common non-immunological cause of pancreatic graft loss (between 5 to 10% for most centres).[14,28,29] There are many factors that contribute to the risk of arterial or venous thrombosis:[27,28]

- Donor factors, such as increasing donor age, cardiocerebrovascular cause of death, haemodynamic instability, substantial fluid resuscitation.
- Retrieval factors, such as suboptimal surgical pancreas retrieval, preservation and backtable preparation, prolonged cold ischaemia time, portal vein extension grafts, arterial reconstructions other than y-graft reconstructions.
- Recipient factors, such as PAK and PTA greater risk than SPK,* enteric drainage greater risk than bladder drainage,* peritoneal dialysis greater risk than haemodialysis, segmental pancreas transplant greater risk than whole organ transplant, left-sided placement greater risk than right-sided placement, hypercoaguable recipients, and post-perfusion graft pancreatitis.

In a previously functioning pancreatic graft, clinical presentations of graft thrombosis include: unexplained hyperglycaemia (arterial and/or venous thrombosis), haematuria (venous thrombosis), abdominal pain, and swelling over the graft side (venous thrombosis).[28] In pancreatic grafts that are bladder-drained a sudden decrease or absence of urinary amylase can occur.

---

*Possibly due to the difficulty associated with early diagnosis of rejection, as neither serum creatinine in PAK and PTA recipients (as there is no same donor, simultaneous kidney transplant), nor urinary amylase with enteric drainage can be monitored.

Imaging studies (duplex Doppler ultrasonography, angiography or CT angiography) can be used to confirm the diagnosis.[14,28]

The diagnosis of graft thrombosis usually results in a graft pancreatectomy. Pharmacological, surgical and percutaneous interventional attempts to salvage thrombosed grafts remain areas of interest, with various techniques, degrees of success and levels of thrombosis.

6.10.1 Bleeding

Intra-abdominal haemorrhage is a common cause of relaparotomy. However, minor bleeding can be managed conservatively with blood transfusions and correction of coagulopathy. It is thought to be responsible for the loss of a graft in 0.3 to 1.5% of all pancreas transplants.[28]

6.10.2 Intra-abdominal infections

Intra-abdominal infections cause a high morbidity and mortality as well as significantly affecting graft survival.[10,14,21] They are associated with an anastomotic leak in 30% of cases. Risk factors include old age (donor and/or recipient), prolonged cold ischaemic time, vascular graft thrombosis and retransplantation over primary transplantation.[21,28] Over 50% of cases result in a graft pancreatectomy.[10]

6.10.3 Graft pancreatitis

Early post-transplant prolonged hyperamylasaemia has been observed in up to 35% of pancreas transplant recipients and thought to be associated with graft pancreatitis in combination with symptoms of abdominal pain and distension and imaging studies (CT or ultrasonography) showing evidence of pancreatic oedema, inflammation and necrosis.[28] Risk factors related to development of graft pancreatitis include prolonged cold ischaemic time, donor factors (such as age, BMI, haemodynamic instability, vasopressor administration), excessive flush volume or pressure on procurement, and in grafts that are bladder drained, reflux pancreatitis secondary to urinary retention.[27,28] Complications of graft pancreatitis include pancreatic necrosis (sterile or infected), perigraft infection, pancreatic abscess, and pancreatic pseudocysts.[28] Octreotide, a somatostatin analogue, is commonly used in the prevention and treatment of graft pancreatitis.[28]

6.10.4 Anastomotic leak

Anastomotic leaks are responsible for 1.5 to 2% of pancreatic graft loss in enteric-drained grafts, and 0.6 to 0.8% of bladder-drained grafts.[2,10] This difference is due to leaks from enteric-drained grafts leaking in the abdominal cavity leading to intra-abdominal sepsis and peritonitis, whereas bladder-drained grafts are associated with a lower infection rate.[10,28–30] Early anastomotic leaks are usually due to technical complications or ischaemia and late leaks are more likely to be due to infection, rejection or ischaemia.[10,14] Clinically, these patients present with abdominal pain, distension, fever and hyperamylasaemia.[28] Management usually requires a relaparotomy and revision of anastomosis or graft pancreatectomy for enteric-drained grafts. Bladder-drained grafts can be managed conservatively, by decompression with a Foley catheter and drainage of intra-abdominal collections in the absence of intra-abdominal infection.[10,28,30]

Other typical complications from major abdominal surgery have been reported in pancreas transplantation including bowel obstruction, prolonged ileus, superficial and deep wound infection, and fascial dehiscence.[2,28]

6.11 The Future

Transplantation of pancreatic tissue is a treatment option for patients with labile diabetes. Currently, whole organ pancreas transplantation is the gold standard and in the future may be the treatment of choice in those who develop diabetes, before they develop diabetic complications. There has been a significant improvement in patient survival and graft outcome in pancreas transplantation over the last several years, with a patient survival rate of 95% at 1 year and 90% at 3 years.[10] In SPK recipients the graft survival rate at 1 year is 85%, reaching almost 80% at 3 years.[10] This is higher than for the other two categories of pancreas transplantation (79% at 1 year), but there has been significant improvement in their outcomes (their greatest problems continue to be immunogenic graft loss, 6% at 1 year for PTA and

PKA compared to 2% for SPK patients).[10] The immediate future of whole organ pancreas transplantation will be to improve on certain key areas:

- The donor pool, by using more marginal organs.
- Preservation: finding the optimum preservation solution; machine organ perfusion.
- Surgical technique.
- Immunosuppression.
- Markers of rejection to aid earlier diagnosis, especially in solitary pancreas transplants.
- Imaging of the graft.

Other strategies employed to try and achieve the goal of insulin independence in these patients include islet cell transplantation, stem cell transplantation, gene therapy live donors and bio-hybrid artificial device units.[31,32]

In the long term, any or all of these strategies may have an important role.

References

1. Nathan, D.M. (1993). The Effect of Intensive Treatment of Diabetes on the Development and Progression of Long-Term Complications in Insulin-Dependent Diabetes Mellitus, *New Engl J Med*, **329**, 977–986.
2. Smith, R.F.P. (2010). 'Indications, Patient Evaluation, and Selection', in Hakim, N. *et al.* (eds.), *Pancreas, Islet and Stem Cell Transplantation for Diabetes*, Second Edition, Oxford University Press, New York, pp. 51–62.
3. Han, D.J. and Sutherland, D.E. (2010). Pancreas Transplantation, *Gut Liver*, **4(4)**, 450–465.
4. Sener, A., Cooper, M. and Bartlett, S.T. (2010). Is There a Role for Pancreas Transplantation in Type 2 Diabetes Mellitus? *Transplantation*, **90(2)**, 121–123.
5. Larsen, J.L. (2004). Pancreas Transplantation: Indications and Consequences, *Endocr Rev*, **25(6)**, 919–946.
6. White, S.A., Shaw, J.A. and Sutherland, D.E. (2009). Pancreas Transplantation, *Lancet*, **373(9677)**, 1808–1817.
7. Iwanaga, Y. *et al.* (2008). Pancreas Preservation for Pancreas and Islet Transplantation, *Curr Opin Organ Transplant*, **13(2)**, 135–141.
8. Brockmann, J.G. *et al.* (2006). Retrieval of Abdominal Organs for Transplantation, *Br J Surg*, **93(2)**, 133–146.
9. Hakim, N. *et al.* (2010). 'Procurement and Benchwork Preparation of the Pancreatic Graft', in Hakim, N. *et al.* (eds.), *Pancreas, Islet and Stem*

Cell Transplantation for Diabetes, Second Edition, Oxford University Press, New York, pp. 85–92.

10. Lam, V.W. *et al.* (2010). Evolution of Pancreas Transplant Surgery, *ANZ J Surg*, **80(6)**, 411–418.

11. Ridgway, D. *et al.* (2010). Preservation of the Donor Pancreas for Whole Pancreas and Islet Transplantation, *Clin Transplant*, **24(1)**, 1–19.

12. Fridell, J.A., Rogers, J. and Stratta, R.J. (2010). The Pancreas Allograft Donor: Current Status, Controversies, and Challenges for the Future, *Clin Transplant*, **24(4)**, 433–449.

13. Boggi, U. *et al.* (2010). 'Surgical Techniques of Pancreas Transplantation', in Hakim, N., Stratta, R.J, Gray, D. *et al.* (eds), *Pancreas, Islet and Stem Cell Transplantation for Diabetes*, Second Edition, Oxford University Press, New York, pp. 111–136.

14. Richter, A., Lerner, S. and Schroppel, B. (2011). Current State of Combined Kidney and Pancreas Transplantation, *Blood Purif*, **31(1–3)**, 96–101.

15. Singh, R.P. and Stratta, R.J. (2008). Advances in Immunosuppression for Pancreas Transplantation, *Curr Opin Organ Transplant*, **13(1)**, 79–84.

16. Gruessner, A.C., Sutherland, D.E. and Gruessner, R.W. (2010). Pancreas Transplantation in the United States. A Review, *Curr Opin Organ Transplant*, **15(1)**, 93–101.

17. Mineo, D. *et al.* (2009). Minimization and Withdrawal of Steroids in Pancreas and Islet Transplantation, *Transpl Int*, **22(1)**, 20–37.

18. Nakache, R., Malaise, J. and Van Ophem, D. (2005). A Large, Prospective, Randomized, Open-Label, Multicentre Study of Corticosteroid Withdrawal in SPK Transplantation: A 3 Year Report, *Nephrol Dial Transplant*, **20(Suppl 2)**, ii40–47, ii62.

19. Gruessner, A.C. and Sutherland, D.E. (2008). Pancreas Transplant Outcomes for United States (US) Cases as Reported to the United Network for Organ Sharing (UNOS) and the International Pancreas Transplant Registry (IPTR), *Clin Transplant*, pp. 45–56.

20. Michalak, G. *et al.* (2005). Surgical Complications of Simultaneous Pancreas-Kidney Transplantation: A 16-Year-Experience at One Center. *Transplant Proc*, **37(8)**, 3555–3557.

21. Martins, L. *et al.* (2010). Pancreas-Kidney Transplantation: Complications and Readmissions in 9 Years of Follow-up, *Transplant Proc*, **42(2)**, 552–554.

22. Sollinger, H.W. *et al.* (2009). One Thousand Simultaneous Pancreas-Kidney Transplants at a Single Center With 22-Year Follow-Up, *Ann Surg*, **250(4)**, 618–630.

23. 2009 Annual Report of the US Organ Procurement and Transplantation Network and the Scientific Registry of Transplant Recipients: Transplant Data 1994–2008. Department of Health and Human Services, Health Resources and Services Administration, Healthcare Systems Bureau, Division

of Transplantation, Rockville, MD; United Network for Organ Sharing, Richmond, VA; University Renal Research and Education Association, Ann Arbor, MI.*

24. Gruessner, A.C. and Sutherland, D.E. (2005). Pancreas Transplant Outcomes for United States (US) and Non-US Cases as Reported to the United Network for Organ Sharing (UNOS) and the International Pancreas Transplant Registry (IPTR) as of June 2004, *Clin Transplant*, **19(4)**, 433–455.

25. Sutherland, D.E. *et al.* (2001). Lessons Learned from More than 1,000 Pancreas Transplants at a Single Institution, *Ann Surg*, **233(4)**, 463–501.

26. Ziaja, J. *et al.* (2009). Impact of Pancreas Transplantation on the Quality of Life of Diabetic Renal Transplant Recipients, *Transplant Proc*, **41(8)**, 3156–3158.

27. Sousa, M.G. *et al.* (2010). Multivariate Analysis of Risk Factors for Early Loss of Pancreas Grafts Among Simultaneous Pancreas-Kidney Transplants, *Transplant Proc*, **42(2)**, 547–551.

28. Troppmann, C. (2010). Complications After Pancreas Transplantation, *Curr Opin Organ Transplant*, **15(1)**, 112–118.

29. Malaise, J. *et al.* (2005). Simultaneous Pancreas-Kidney Transplantation in a Large Multicenter Study: Surgical Complications, *Transplant Proc*, **37(6)**, 2859–2860.

30. Sansalone, C.V. *et al.* (2005). Surgical Complications are the Main Cause of Pancreatic Allograft Loss in Pancreas-Kidney Transplant Recipients, *Transplant Proc*, **37(6)**, 2651–2653.

31. Vardanyan, M. *et al.* (2010). Pancreas vs. Islet Transplantation: A Call on the Future, *Curr Opin Organ Transplant*, **15(1)**, 124–130.

32. Rowinski, W. (2007). Future of Transplantation Medicine, *Ann Transplant*, **12(1)**, 5–10.

*This work was supported in part by Health Resources and Services Administration contract 234-2005-37011C. The content is the responsibility of the authors alone and does not necessarily reflect the views or policies of the Department of Health and Human Services, nor does mention of trade names, commercial products, or organizations imply endorsement by the US Government.

7

Liver Transplantation

Madhava Pai and Ruben Canelo

7.1 Introduction

Liver transplantation (LT) has been an accepted treatment for end-stage liver disease since the 1980s. It has undergone a revolutionary change since its first clinical application in 1963, when Thomas Starzl at the University of Colorado first attempted liver replacement in a three-year-old boy with biliary atresia; the procedure, however, could not be completed due to massive haemorrhage.[1] During the next few years, several more attempts at liver replacement were not successful in the long term. The introduction of azathioprine and antilymphocyte serum in the mid 1960s helped to overcome some of the problems. In 1967, Tom Starzl replaced the liver of an 18-month-old girl with primary hepatocellular carcinoma, who lived for 13 months before dying of diffuse metastases.[2] Throughout the 1970s, two teams — one in Colorado led by Tom Starzl[3] and the other in Cambridge led by Sir Roy Calne[4] — continued their efforts at clinical liver transplantation.

Along with the clinical introduction of cyclosporine by Calne in 1978,[5] improvements in surgical techniques, donor and recipient selection criteria, perioperative care, and use of the venous bypass[6–8] stimulated worldwide enthusiasm for liver transplantation. Cyclosporine improved the one-year survival rate from 33% to over 70% for the first 67 patients treated by Starzl's

125

group between 1980 and 1982.[9] In the late 1980s, yet another advance was the development of the University of Wisconsin (UW) solution for organ allograft preservation. UW solution has extended the safe cold storage time from a previous maximum of 8 hours to the current maximum of 24 hours.[10–15] It has changed LT from an emergency to a semi-elective procedure, and made more distant procurement possible. Prolonged preservation time has also allowed the development of reduced-size, split-liver, and auxiliary liver transplantation.[16,17]

In the last few decades, considerable progress has been made in the care of liver transplant candidates and recipients. At present, the one- and five-year patient survival rates are approximately 85 and 75%, respectively.[18] Although outcomes after transplantation have improved enormously, this has been largely incremental. Improvements not only in surgical techniques but also in recipient selection, donor management and selection, anaesthesia, and postoperative care, as well as advances in understanding of the microbiology and better usage and a greater spectrum of immunosuppressive agents, have raised survival results over the years. Although advances in surgical techniques have effectively increased the donor pool, the increase in donor organs has not kept pace with the increasing demand. Currently, LT is the treatment of choice for acute and chronic liver failure.

7.2 Indications

In the early years, patients were only referred for a transplant at the terminal stage of their liver disease. But with the improved patient and graft survival rates, liver transplantation has emerged as the optimal therapy for patients with end-stage liver disease.[19–21] The recent years are characterized by a considerable broadening as well as a progressively changing pattern of liver transplant indications. Although in the past cancers constituted up to 50% of all the indications for transplants, currently this indication accounts for 13 to 15%. The same trait has been observed among patients with primary biliary cirrhosis (PBC), whose numbers have been decreasing, as opposed to the increasing number of patients transplanted for alcoholic and hepatitis C cirrhosis, who currently represent the most common indications for LT in Europe and the United States.[18,22]

Based on the most recent European Liver Transplant Registry (ELTR) report,[18] in adult patients, cirrhosis accounts for the majority of transplants performed (58%), with alcoholism (18%) and hepatitis C (15%) being the two most common underlying conditions. Other transplant indications include cholestatic liver diseases (PBC and primary sclerosing cholangitis [PSC]), metabolic diseases (Wilson's disease, familial amyloidotic polyneuropathy [FAP], α-1 antitrypsin deficiency), and chronic hepatitis (hepatitis B, autoimmune). Transplants are also performed for liver cancers (13%). Although LT is reserved predominantly for nonmetastatic hepatocellular carcinoma (HCC) (9%), other tumor types (primary and secondary) are currently treated with transplant surgery. Patients transplanted for acute hepatic failure make up 9% of total transplants. The main causes of acute hepatic failure are acute viral hepatitis and drug toxicity (predominantly acetaminophen).

Pediatric LTs account for 10% of all liver transplants performed so far by the European transplant programs.[18] The predominant indication for transplant is cholestatic liver disease, representing 73% of all the indications in pediatric patients aged 0 to 2 years old, and 43% of the indications in patients aged 2 to 15 years old. Metabolic disease is the second most common indication (10% for patients aged 0 to 2 years, and 26% for patients aged 2 to 15 years). In the metabolic group of indications, the most common condition is α-1 antitrypsin deficiency, followed by cholestatic disorders such as Alagille syndrome and sclerosing cholangitis (Table 7.1).

End-stage liver disease secondary to hepatitis B is a common indication for liver transplantation. The post-transplant recurrence rate is as high as 100%.[23-28] With the limited number of donor organs available, controversy exists as to whether these patients should receive liver transplants.[29-31] Patients with active hepatitis B viral replication at the time of their transplant are at greater risk for recurrence.[32] Patient and graft survival rates profoundly decrease for recipients with post-transplant recurrent hepatitis B, because the recurrent form takes on a more virulent and aggressive course, leading to fatal liver failure in one to two years.

Hepatitis C remains a particularly difficult problem because nearly all patients develop disease recurrence after LT, which has an adverse outcome in the graft and overall survival rates.[33,34] Survival after retransplant for recurrent hepatitis C is poor, and retransplant for these patients remains

Table 7.1 Indications for liver
transplantation.

Adults
Chronic active hepatitis B
Chronic active hepatitis C
Alcoholic cirrhosis
Primary biliary cirrhosis
Primary sclerosing cholangitis
Metabolic disorders
Neoplasms
Fulminant hepatitis
Autoimmune hepatitis
Trauma

Children
Biliary atresia or hypoplasia
Metabolic disorders
Neonatal hepatitis
Fulminant hepatitis
Neoplasms

controversial.[34,35] Hepatitis C has been shown to have a recurrence rate of
88 to 100% in the transplanted liver.[23,24,30] However, its course is usually
much less devastating than a post-transplant hepatitis B infection, many
patients having clinically silent disease. The course is milder in spite of
increased post-transplant hepatitis C viral replication.[36] Many variables are
likely to be involved, including the level of pre-transplant viremia, genotype
of the virus, amount of post-transplant immunosuppression, and ability of
the host immune system to recognize the hepatitis C virus and mount an
immune response.[30]

   Alcoholic liver disease (ALD) is one of the most common indications for
LT and has similar short- and long-term survival results as nonalcoholic-
related causes of cirrhosis.[18,22] Recipients with alcohol-related disease have
a surprisingly low rate of recidivism if carefully selected. Selection criteria
includes a period of abstinence, enrollment in a treatment program before
and after transplantation, recognition and acknowledgment by the patient

of his or her problem with alcohol, a commitment by the patient to abstain from alcohol, and a good social support system. The majority of transplant centers (85%) use a period of six months of abstinence before considering patients for LT.[37]

Liver transplantation can cure as many as 30% (at five years) of patients with hepatic malignancies who would otherwise die of their disease.[38,39] Controversy continues to exist as to whether organs should instead be given to recipients with nonmalignant liver disease.[40,41] Indications for early transplantation include rapid deterioration of liver function, hepatic encephalopathy, deterioration in hepatic synthetic function, and hepatic osteodystrophia. In such patients, liver replacement is urgent before metabolic acidosis, septicemia, and multiple organ failure develop. Transjugular intrahepatic portosystemic shunt (TIPS) placement in patients who have variceal bleeding or refractory ascites decreases episodes of variceal hemorrhage, operative transfusion requirements, operative time, and length of hospital stay; it increases graft and patient survival.[42,43] However, it also increases the risk of portal vein thrombosis as well as the incidence of encephalopathy. At present, patients should be referred for a transplant when they experience a late complication of their chronic liver disease, develop decompensation of previously stable liver disease, or suffer significant impairment in their quality of life directly related to their liver disease.[44] Early referral is the key to a successful liver transplant.

7.3 Contraindications

For all patients with advanced liver disease, critical issues include determining contraindications, interpreting pre-transplant work-up results, and properly timing the transplant. Although contraindications have changed over the years, they still include extrahepatic malignancy, sepsis, and active substance abuse (Table 7.2).[44] Surgical risk should be assessed by general evaluation of cardiac, pulmonary, and renal function; in addition, previous complications and operations must be considered, as well as the nature and stage of the underlying liver disease. The pre-transplant work-up should determine not only if a patient requires a transplant, but also how urgently.

Table 7.2 Contraindications to liver transplantation.

Absolute
Extrahepatic malignancy
Hepatic malignancy with diffuse tumor invasion
Untreated sepsis
Active drug or alcohol abuse
Advanced cardiopulmonary disease

Relative
HIV
Age
Portal venous thrombosis
Previous malignancy
Active psychiatric illness
Cholangiocarcinoma

According to the 2007 ELTR report, the proportion of patients over 60 years of age transplanted in Europe has significantly increased in the past 15 years, currently constituting more than 20% of the transplanted patients as opposed to 10% in the mid 1990s.[18] Another condition that not so long ago was considered an absolute contraindication to LT is human immunodeficiency virus (HIV) infection. The introduction of highly active antiretroviral therapy (HAART) has greatly improved the survival of these patients.[45,46] Similarly, evolving treatment strategies have changed the approach toward cholangiocarcinoma, which is still considered by many centers as an absolute contraindication. The results found by Sudan *et al.* (one- and five-year survival rates of 88% and 82%, respectively) have shown that an aggressive approach using a combination of radiotherapy and chemotherapy with surgery can identify a proportion of patients who will eventually benefit from LT.[47]

7.4 Organ Allocation

The multidisciplinary teams (consisting of surgeons, hepatologists, anesthetists, coordinators, and social workers) decide about the indication and patient's suitability for LT. Approval by the multidisciplinary team leads to adding the patient to the LT waiting list. Prioritization of patients while waiting for LT is dynamic and changes over time depending on their clinical status. Presently, the highest priority for organ allocation is given to patients with fulminant hepatic failure (FHF). Although selection criteria in the setting of FHF are not yet standardized, King's College Hospital or Clichy criteria are the most commonly used (depending on centers' preference) to predict the outcome and assess the need for LT.[48,49]

Elective patients are considered for LT in a descending order based on their model for end-stage liver disease (MELD) or pediatric end-stage liver disease (PELD) score. The latter is used for patients up to 12 years. In the United States, where the model of organ allocation is patient-based, the MELD score has been used since 2002.[22] The principle behind using the MELD score is the "sickest first" policy, in which not the time on the waiting list but the risk of mortality is the determining factor in deciding the organ allocation.

The change to the MELD system has been extremely successful, resulting in a reduction in medial waiting time and mortality while on the waiting list and unchanged early graft and patient survival as compared with the previous allocation systems. Originally developed to calculate the risk for survival after placement of a TIPS, the MELD score proved to be a predictor of survival in various liver diseases.[50] The score is obtained by a mathematical calculation using three widely available laboratory variables: international normalized ratio (INR), serum creatinine, and serum bilirubin. The calculation is:

$$MELD = 9.57 \times \log e \, (\text{creatinine}) + 3.78 \times \log e \, (\text{total bilirubin})$$
$$+ 11.2 \times \log (INR) + 6.43.$$

7.5 Donor Selection

The progress made in the field of LT has led physicians to offer it to an increasingly complex population with an increasing success rate. However, at the same time, the availability of cadaveric organs has diminished, resulting in the number of potential candidates exceeding organ supply with attendant deaths on the waiting list. With the expanding recipient indications, LT has become a victim of its own success. Despite intense educational efforts to increase consent for donation, the number of organ donors has remained relatively constant. As a result, many centers selectively accept liver grafts from the so-called extended-criteria donors. There is still no clear definition of extended criteria, but donors are considered marginal if there is a risk of initial poor function or primary nonfunction. Generally, extended donor criteria are divided into donor specific (age over 65 years, steatosis greater than 30% of graft volume, long interval between brain death and procurement, or graft infected by hepatitis B or C) and procurement specific (cold ischemia greater than 12 hours).

As shown by ELTR data, donors older than 50 years currently provide more than 20% of the transplanted liver grafts.[18] Similarly, United Network for Organ Sharing (UNOS) data show that cadaveric donors older than 50 years accounted for 25% of all transplanted livers in 1996 and the number increased to 34% in 2006.[22] The increased risk associated with steatosis is mainly restricted with severe macrosteatosis (>60%), hence these livers should not be used. In contrast, livers with mild macrosteatosis (<30%) are increasingly being used by transplant centers with very good results. Good results have been reported with the use of hepatitis C-positive grafts for hepatitis C-infected patients.[51] Provided the donor liver is not fibrotic, survival after transplant can be unimpaired. A report based on UNOS data showed that the two-year survival rate was significantly higher in hepatitis C virus (HCV)-positive patients who received HCV-positive grafts compared with HCV-positive patients who received HCV-negative grafts.[52]

Prolonged cold ischemia is a very important, independent factor because it is directly related not only to primary nonfunction (PNF) but also to patient and graft survival.[53] As demonstrated by Adam et al., cold ischemia for longer than 12 hours has been associated with a twofold increase in preservation damage, resulting in prolonged post-operative course, biliary tract strictures, and decreased graft survival.[54–56]

A careful review of the donor history is the first step for overall assessment. Once the donor history has been reviewed, laboratory values are more meaningful and trends are easier to interpret. No standardized criteria can clearly predict whether the donor liver will provide good function. The final decision should be based on the donor surgeon's impression after inspection of the liver at the time of procurement, combined with histologic quantification of the proportion of macrovesicular fat.[40] Hepatic trauma, evidence of early cirrhosis, marked edema, and speckled or marbled liver surface, are all generally considered poor prognostic signs. Because of the current organ shortage the subject of non-heart-beating donors is being revisited.[57,58]

7.6 Donor Hepatectomy

In the multi-organ procurement technique, the abdomen and thorax are entered through a complete midline sternal-splitting incision.[59] Before the actual dissecting begins, it is important to identify all variations of hepatic arterial supply. Aberrant branches to the right lobe arise from the superior mesenteric artery and pass behind the common duct and portal vein to the right lobe. Aberrant branches to the left lobe take off the left gastric artery, and therefore the gastrohepatic ligament must be inspected and palpated. All atypical branches must be carefully preserved. After the arterial blood supply to the liver is identified, a Kocher maneuver of the duodenum is performed, the common duct is divided, and the gallbladder drained; the hepatic artery and celiac axis origin are dissected free, the suspensory ligaments of the liver are divided, and the supra- and infrahepatic vena cava are mobilized and encircled. Once the dissection of liver, pancreas, and kidneys is completed, cannulas are inserted in the aorta, infrarenal cava, and portal vein. Then the preservation solution is infused. With the use of non heart beating donors, en bloc resection of the abdominal organs has been advocated.[57,60] These organs are then separated on the back table.

7.7 Recipient Operation

In many cases, the most difficult part of the liver replacement is the recipient hepatectomy. Previous surgery on hepatic hilar structures or portal hypertension may result in massive bleeding. The use of cell saver and pump-driven venovenous bypass systems during the recipient hepatectomy and the anhepatic phase of the operation have significantly reduced mortality.[59] Another factor that has decreased perioperative mortality in recent years is the improved resuscitative management by anesthesia teams, including substitution of blood loss and correction of coagulopathy, electrolyte shifts, hypoxemia, and hypothermia. A bilateral subcostal incision with a midline

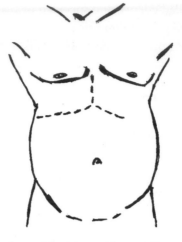

Figure 7.1 A bilateral subcostal incision with a midline extension to the xiphoid is used, extending more on the right than on the left.

extension to the xiphoid is used, extending more on the right than on the left (Figure 7.1). Once the native liver is removed, first the suprahepatic vena cava is anastomosed, then the infrahepatic vena cava. According to the Minnesota liver replacement technique, the portal bypass cannula is then removed and the portal vein is reconstructed.[59] The liver is then revascularized with portal flow; the clamp on the suprahepatic vena cava, however, is not released. Venous backflow from the mesentery is flushed via the partially sutured anterior wall of the infrahepatic caval anastomosis to avoid release of cold, acidotic, and hyperkalemic preservation fluid into the circulation, which could cause pulmonary artery vasoconstriction and subsequent hypotension. After the anterior wall of the infrahepatic vena cava is closed, the hepatic artery is reconstructed. Direct anastomosis of the donor to the recipient hepatic artery is always desirable, but often not feasible because of size discrepancy, variations in both donor and recipient liver arteries, or injury of the native artery. In these cases, alternative methods of vascular reconstruction must be used.[59] Finally, the biliary system is reconstructed with a direct duct-to-duct reconstruction; either end-to-side or side-to-side over a T-tube is preferred (Figure 7.2). In patients with diseases of the extrahepatic biliary system, a Roux-en-Y anastomosis (choledochojejunostomy) over a stent is performed. Intraoperatively, satisfactory liver graft function is

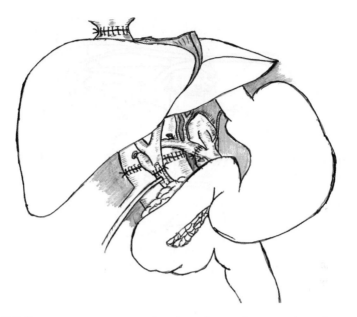

Figure 7.2 Post anastomoses: completed caval, portal venous, hepatic arterial and biliary anastomoses.

manifested by early restoration of clotting function and appearance of bile in the drainage catheter.

An alternative method of liver transplantation is the piggyback operation.[61,62] In this method the recipient inferior vena cava (IVC) is left intact (Figure 7.3). The branches of the IVC to the liver, except the hepatic veins, are suture ligated. Doing so allows a partial occluding clamp to be placed on the vena cava. It preserves caval blood flow to the heart, minimizing the hemodynamic disturbances of total IVC clamping. With this technique, venous–venous bypass is sometimes avoided. Many centers use this technique in children.

Before the IVC clamp is released the liver is flushed with portal venous blood. Doing so avoids retrocaval dissection, helps adjust for size disparities between the donor and recipient vessels, ensures better control of the adrenal vein, and preserves the entire recipient IVC.[61] During the split-liver or living-related liver transplant, the recipient vena cava is usually left intact (the piggyback technique). The donor graft is often the left lobe, or more commonly the left lateral segment.[63–66] Vascular reconstruction is done end

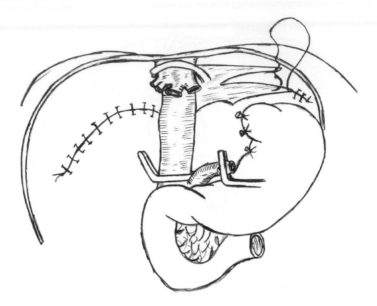

Figure 7.3 Piggyback operation: the liver excised off the retro hepatic cava, leaving the entire vessel in place.

to end or end to side for the left hepatic vein, and end to end for the portal vein. The left hepatic artery anastomosis is to the proper hepatic artery or to the infrarenal aorta by extension graft. During auxiliary liver transplantation, again, a segmental graft is used. The recipient procedure consists of a left-lobe resection. The graft may be placed in an orthotopic or heterotopic position. This method is for patients with acute or subacute hepatic failure and metabolic liver disease. After the recipient's liver recovers, the segment can be removed or the immunosuppression can be stopped.[17]

Over the years many centers have abandoned the routine use of venous–venous bypass.[67] Selective criteria for the use of venous–venous bypass at these centers include patients that cannot tolerate the decreased venous return with vena caval clamping, or are hemodynamically unstable at the beginning of the procedure.[68] Still, others feel that venovenous bypass that precedes the dissection of the vena cava, and bare area of the liver decreases blood loss, and operative time, especially in a patient with significant portal hypertension.[40] Due to the shortage of suitably sized donor organs, especially for infants and small children with end-stage liver disease, three approaches have been developed in recent years: reduced-size orthotopic liver transplantation, split-liver transplantation, and living-related donor liver transplantation.

In reduced-size orthotopic liver transplantation, an anatomic dissection is performed, usually providing the smaller left lobe or lateral segment for transplantation.[17,63] Reduced-size transplantation has redistributed the donor pool to small recipients and decreased the waiting time for children; however, it does not help with the overall shortage of donor organs. Therefore, split-liver transplantation has been attempted, but its use accounts only for 3% of the transplants done in the United States[22] and 5% in Europe.[18] As of 2007, 3,523 cases have been performed by European transplant centers, resulting in a five-year graft survival rate of 62%.[18] Left-split grafts transplanted in children and right-trisegmental grafts transplanted in adults have produced good outcomes.

7.7.1 Domino liver grafts (DLT)

The livers of some selected LT recipients can, in turn, be used for transplanting in another patient. This method, known as domino LT (DLT), is another strategy used by an increasing number of centers.

7.8 Living Donor Liver Transplantation

Living donor liver transplantation (LDLT) is a surgical method in which a partial liver graft is obtained from a living donor and transplanted into a recipient. Since the first successful LDLT by Strong in 1989,[69] this technique has become the primary liver transplant procedure in Asia where an extreme shortage of organs from deceased donors exists due to cultural issues in this geographic region. Furthermore, LDLT has also emerged as an adjunct transplant option in countries with low donation rates. LDLT has become an especially important option for the treatment of pediatric patients, as well as for adult patients who are otherwise disadvantaged by the current allocation system. The method clearly offers the advantage of reducing a patient's time on the waiting list. The reported overall rate of complications ranges from 9 to 67%,[70,71] whereas the mortality rate ranges from 0.05% (left lobe) to 0.4 to 0.5% (right lobe).[72,73] Following the mortality events in the

United States, mandating LDLT guidelines have been created for transplant surgeons.[74]

7.8.1 Minimal graft volume and small–for–size syndrome

One of the most important issues in LDLT is obtaining a minimal viable graft volume because below a certain threshold the partial graft cannot sustain metabolic, synthetic, and detoxifying functions. In cases when the graft is too small, the patient develops clinical signs of liver failure and, later, life–threatening multiorgan failure. This clinical feature is termed a "small–for–size syndrome (SFSS)."[75,76] To prevent SFSS, an allograft volume of 35 to 40% of a normal liver or a graft–to–total–body–weight ratio of 0.8 to 1% must be obtained.[77]

7.9 Immunosuppression

The majority of centers uses a triple combination immunosuppressive regimen, including calcineurin inhibitors (CNIs), corticosteroids, and antimetabolite drugs.

7.9.1 Induction therapy

Current trends in the United States show that interleukin (IL)-2 receptor antibodies are commonly used compared with other agents (ornithine-ketoacid transaminase orthoclone [OKT3], antithymocyte globulin [ATG]); however, there is little evidence to advocate one treatment over the other.[78]

7.9.2 Maintenance therapy

The standard maintenance regimen is based on corticosteroids (prednisolone), CNIs (cyclosporine A [CsA] or tacrolimus), and antimetabolites (mycophenolate mofetil [MMF] or azathioprine). Corticosteroids are generally used after LT. Although there has been a trend toward rapid steroid reduction and withdrawal shortly after transplant (within days),[79,80] most patients are discharged with oral steroid, which is completely withdrawn over a few months after LT, leaving the CNIs as the mainstay immunosuppressive agents in 95% of cases.[22] The CNIs (CsA and tacrolimus) remain the cornerstones of the immunosuppressive therapies in most transplant centers. Nevertheless, the use of CsA can be associated with side effects such as nephrotoxicity, dyslipidemia, and hypertension. Although the tacrolimus therapy has been shown to be associated with a lower incidence of hypertension and hyperlipidemia, it has the same nephrotoxicity and has a higher incidence rate of diabetes and neurotoxicity.

MMF is as safe as azathioprine. Also, several studies, including a large multicenter trial, have shown that the use of MMF in combination with either tacrolimus or CsA has proved to be very effective in reducing the incidence of acute cellular rejection as well as in allowing steroid withdrawal and CNI reduction.[80] The new potent immunosuppressive drugs sirolimus and everolimus (mTOR inhibitors) are still being evaluated.

7.10 Complications After Liver Transplantation

7.10.1 Liver-related causes of morbidity and mortality

7.10.1.1 *Recurrence of disease*

Recurrence of hepatocellular carcinoma is especially common in patients with a poorly differentiated tumor or macroscopic vascular invasion.[81] Surgical treatment of recurrent disease should be considered, but outcome is almost universally dismal.[82] Recurrence of autoimmune disease in an organ from a donor is immunologically intriguing. Diagnosis can be difficult due to other potential causes for graft dysfunction. Recurrence of an early stage of PBC may occur in a majority of patients transplanted for this indication in the long term, but seldom leads to cirrhosis.[83] Recurrence of autoimmune hepatitis is seen in 22% of patients, and is treated as in nontransplant patients.[84] Recurrence of PSC occurs in about 11% of patients;[84] diagnosis may be difficult because of overlap with nonanastomotic strictures from other causes.

7.10.1.2 *Biliary complications*

Biliary complications are an important source of morbidity, and in severe cases even loss of the graft or mortality. Despite great improvements in both surgical and medical management of liver transplant recipients, biliary complications are still common, occurring in 6 to 35% of patients.[85] It appears that the biliary epithelium is much more susceptible to ischaemic injury than liver parenchyma and gross vascular structures.[86] The biliary anastomosis in liver transplantation is most commonly performed making an end-to-end anastomosis of the donor and recipient common bile duct (choledochoc- holedochostomy or duct-to-duct anastomosis). The remainder of transplants are performed using a Roux-en-Y anastomosis (hepaticojejunostomy), espe- cially when the recipient bile duct is too short or unsuitable, i.e., in patients with primary sclerosing cholangitis.

Of the biliary complications, leakage of bile and strictures of the biliary tree are most commonly encountered. Bile leakage is usually seen shortly after transplantation and occurs in 5 to 7% of patients.[85] It can occur at the site of the anastomosis, the cystic duct remnant or at the exit site of a biliary drain. The majority of cases can be successfully managed by placement of a stent through the sphincter of Oddi, reducing pressure in the common bile duct and preventing further leakage.[87,88]

Strictures of the biliary tree can be divided into anastomotic strictures (occurring at the site of the anastomosis of donor and recipients common bile duct) or nonanastomotic strictures (occurring elsewhere in the bil- iary system of the donor liver). Anastomotic strictures are usually due to fibrotic healing, and can be managed by ERCP in the vast majority of cases without any negative effects on the graft or patient survival.[89] Nonanasto- motic strictures (NAS) are of a much more complex nature. They occur in approximately 15% of cases and can present both early and late after transplantation.[90] Their pathogenesis can be immunological, ischaemic or both.[91] In a number of patients, NAS are due to recurrent primary sclerosing cholangitis. In severe cases, NAS can lead to progressive destruction of the biliary tree, causing recurrent bacterial cholangitis, biliary fibrosis or even cirrhosis. Treatment can be attempted with multiple sessions of dilatation and stenting of stenotic areas. A considerable number of patients, however, will need a retransplantation.[92,93]

7.10.2 Liver-unrelated causes of morbidity and mortality

Weight gain and obesity are frequently observed in transplant patients. Obesity usually develops in the first two years post LT, affecting up to 40% of the patients. Causes include steroid use, appetite stimulation by immunosuppressive drugs, and increased sense of well-being. Post-transplant patients have an increased risk of developing cardiovascular disease, which is promoted by several factors (e.g., obesity, diabetes, and hyperlipidemia). The high prevalence of risk factors leads to a markedly increased risk for atherosclerosis and subsequent cardiovascular events. Renal insufficiency is a major cause of morbidity and mortality following LT. The cumulative risk of renal failure has been reported to be as high as 20% at 5 years post transplant. Hypertension, use of CNIs, and pre-transplant renal dysfunction are major contributing factors. Osteoporosis is a common condition in patients post LT. The implicated underlying factors include low calcium and vitamin D, low muscle mass, inactivity, poor nutrition, and prolonged use of steroids. Liver transplant patients have increased risk to develop *de novo* malignancy with an incidence ranging between 5 and 15% in most reported series.[94]

7.10.2.1 *Monitoring for disease recurrence*

Currently, recurrence of hepatitis B is reduced radically by the regular use of antiviral prophylaxis (lamivudine, pegylated interferon) following LT. Also, pre-operative use of antiviral therapies is a factor that has contributed to recurrence reduction, with rates currently at 10%.[95] Hepatitis C, however, is much more difficult to treat. Hepatitis C reinfection is nearly a universal event and is associated with histological changes in 50 to 80% of patients.[33] In contrast to hepatitis B, the antiviral therapies in this group of patients have a modest benefit and also are complicated by several side effects.

7.11 Transplant Outcomes

7.11.1 Overall outcomes

The progress made in transplantation has been associated with significant survival improvements. Based on the 2007 ELTR report, the one-, five-, and ten-year survival rates (all indications combined) are 83%, 71%, and 61%, respectively.[18] Particular survival improvement has been observed in patients transplanted for malignancy whose current one-year survival rate is 89% compared with 79% obtained in the mid 1990s. A similar survival improvement has been observed among patients with cirrhosis (one-year survival of 89%) and also hepatic failure (one-year survival of 78%). Survival improvements have also been observed among pediatric patients. In fact, the five-year survival in children is much better than in adults (78% versus 70%). With regards to retransplantation, the outcomes have been reported to be poor, especially with hepatitis C patients.[34,35] Cumulative data from different studies have shown the following parameters to be strong predictors of survival after retransplant surgery: interval to retransplant, female donor, recipient age, mechanical ventilation, creatinine, total number of grafts, cause of graft failure, and urgency.

7.11.2 Extended criteria and non–heart-beating donors (NHBDs)

The outcome of patients transplanted with grafts obtained from extended criteria donors (ECDs) has been shown to be poor (increased graft loss and decreased survival). In addition, it has been observed that the risk of mortality significantly increases when recipients with advanced age or urgent status are given grafts from ECDs (urgent recipient status increases the risk ratio of death by 50%). Similarly, the use of grafts from NHBDs has also resulted in inferior outcomes.

7.11.3 Living donor

The results of LDLT have been excellent in pediatric recipients of live-donor grafts. Different reports show that the results of LDLT in pediatric patients (children aged under two years) exceed the results of cadaveric grafts.[58–60] Similarly, large series in adult patients have shown that outcomes with LDLT are comparable to those with deceased donor LT (DDLT).[96] In a study by Foster *et al.*, the one- and three-year patient survival and graft survival rates after LDLT were similar to those after DDLT.[97] Overall, however, the potential for recipient complications (biliary, vascular, primary graft nonfunction, and small-for-size graft),[98] as well as donor complications, exists, with an overall donor morbidity rate as high as 29% (with 3.5% of patients experiencing severe complications) and mortality less than 1%.[99] Also, different groups have reported that LDLT is superior to DDLT for patients with HCC within the Milan criteria who wait longer than seven months.[100,101] The current reported mortality rate of a living donor hepatectomy is 0.2 to 0.5%, with a complication rate of 15 to 40%.[102–106] These results are generally more favorable than seen after hepatic resections for malignancy. A recently published series of 335 LDLTs from a single institution in Japan showed four-year graft and recipient survival rate of 66% and 68%, respectively.[105] In this series, the most frequent complication was infection (58%) followed by biliary complications (33%) and acute rejection (33%).

7.11.4 Domino liver grafts (DLT)

Currently, DLT constitutes 1% of the total number of transplantions.[18] Data from the DLT registry (DLTR) has shown overall one-, five-, and eight-year survival rates of 79.9%, 65.3%, and 61.6%, respectively.

7.11.5 Quality of life (QoL)

The evidence so far shows that QoL improves dramatically after LT, compared with health status before transplant surgery. QoL of LT patients is better than or similar to that of the general population.[107] In contrast, a systematic review by Tome *et al.* has demonstrated that although QoL improves after LT, when compared with healthy controls the QoL of LT patients is inferior.[108]

7.12 Summary

Over the past three decades, LT has changed from an experimental procedure with high morbidity to the treatment of choice for patients with end-stage liver disease. Due to standardized operative techniques, improved anesthesia and nursing care, and a better understanding of immunosuppressive drugs, LT has become relatively straightforward. In spite of the improved survival after LT in recent years, the donor organ shortage is especially severe for infants and small children. New technical approaches, such as reduced-size, split-liver, and living-related liver transplantation, may help overcome this shortage. Living-related transplants may also have some immunologic advantage.

References

1. Starzl, T.E. *et al.* (1963). Homotransplantation of the Liver in Humans, *Surg Gynecol Obstet*, **117**, 659–676.
2. Starzl, T.E. *et al.* (1968). Orthotopic Homotransplantation of the Human Liver, *Ann Surg*, **168**, 392–415.
3. Starzl, T.E. *et al.* (1982). Evolution of Liver Transplantation, *Hepatology*, **2**, 614–636.
4. Calne, R.Y. (1987). In: Calne, R.Y. (ed.), *Liver Transplantation: The Cambridge/King's College Hospital Experience*, Second Edition, Grune & Stratton, Orlando, FL, USA, pp. 541–553.
5. Calne, R.Y. *et al.* (1979). Cyclosporin A Initially as the Only Immunosuppressant in 34 Patients of Cadaveric Organs: 32 Kidneys, 2 Pancreases, and 2 Livers, *Lancet*, **2**, 1033–1036.
6. Shaw Jr., B.W. *et al.* (1984). Venous Bypass in Clinical Liver Transplantation, *Ann Surg*, **200**, 524–534.
7. Toledo-Pereyra, L.H. and MacKenzie, G.H. (1983). Orthotopic Liver Transplantation with the Assistance of an External Shunt and a Nonpulsatile Perfusion Pump, *Transplantation*, **35**, 102–104.
8. Griffith, B.P. *et al.* (1985). Venovenous Bypass without Systemic Anticoagulation for Transplantation of the Human Liver, *Surg Gynecol Obstet*, **160**, 270–272.
9. Starzl, T.B. *et al.* (1981). Liver Transplantation with the Use of Cyclosporin A and Prednisone, *New Engl J Med*, **305**, 266–269.
10. Jamieson, N.V. *et al.* (1988). Successful 24- to 30-Hour Preservation of the Canine Liver: A Preliminary Report, *Transplant Proc*, **20**, 945–947.
11. Kalayoglu, M. *et al.* (1988). Extended Preservation of the Liver for Clinical Transplantation, *Lancet*, **1**, 617–619.
12. Belzer, F.O. *et al.* (1992). The Use of UW Solution in Clinical Transplantation. A 4-Year Experience, *Ann Surg*, **2(15)**, 579–583.
13. Blankensteijn, J.D. and Terpstra, O.T. (1991). Liver Preservation: The Past and the Future, *Hepatology*, **13**, 1235–1250.
14. Stratta, R.J. *et al.* (1990). The Impact of Extended Preservation on Clinical Liver Transplantation, *Transplantation*, **50**, 438–443.
15. Todo, S. *et al.* (1989). Extended Preservation of Human Liver Grafts with UW Solution, *JAMA*, **261**, 711–714.
16. Fortner, J.C. *et al.* (1973). Clinical Liver Heterotopic (Auxiliary) Transplantation, *Surgery*, **74**, 739–751.
17. Pappas, S.C., Rouch, D.A. and Stevens, L.H. (1995). New Techniques for Liver Transplantation: Reduced-Size, Split Liver, Living-Related and Auxiliary Liver Transplantation, *Scand J Gastroenterol*, **208**, 97–100.
18. European Liver Transplant Registry. (2007). *Data Analysis Booklet*. Available at: http://www.eltr.org/spip.php?page=documents

19. Busuttil, R.W. *et al.* (1987). The First 100 Liver Transplants at UCLA, *Ann Surg*, **206**, 387–403.
20. Friend, P.J. *et al.* (1989). Liver Transplantation in the Cambridge/King's College Hospital Series—The First 400 Patients, *Transplant Proc*, **21**, 2397–2398.
21. Kilpe, Y.E., Krakauer, H. and Wren, R.E. (1993). An Analysis of Liver Transplant Experience from 37 Transplant Centers as Reported to Medicare, *Transplantation*, **56**, 554–561.
22. United Network for Organ Sharing. *Data Reports*. Available at: http://www.unos.org/donation/index.php?topic=data
23. Heifron, T.G. (1995). Living-Related Liver Transplantation, *Semin Liver Dis*, **15**, 165–172.
24. Gane, E.J. *et al.* (1996). Long-Term Outcome of Hepatitis C Infection after Liver Transplantation, *New Engl J Med*, **334**, 815–820.
25. Randhawa, P.S. and Demetris, A.J. (1995). Hepatitis C Virus Infection in Liver Allografts, *Pathol Annu*, **30**, 203–226.
26. Ringe, B. *et al.* (1995). Recurrence of Hepatitis B Virus Cirrhosis and Hepatocellular Carcinoma: An Indication for Retransplantation? *Clin Transplant*, **9**, 190–196.
27. Langrehr, J.M. *et al.* (1995). Liver Transplantation in Hepatitis B Surface Antigen Positive Patients with Postoperative Long-Term Immunoprophylaxis, *Transplant Proc*, **27**, 1215–1216.
28. Holt, C.D., Millis, J.M. and Busuttil, R.W. (1995). Role of Liver Transplantation in Patients with Hepatitis B Infection, *Clin Transplant*, **9**, 269–276.
29. Demetris, A.J. *et al.* (1990). Evolution of Hepatitis B Virus Liver Disease after Hepatic Replacement: Practical and Theoretical Considerations, *Am J Pathol*, **137**, 667–676.
30. Chazouilleres, O. and Wright, T.L. (1995). Hepatitis C and Liver Transplantation, *J Gastroenterol Hepatol*, **10**, 471–480.
31. Jansen, P. *et al.* (1995). Hepatitis B–Associated Liver Cirrhosis as an Indication for Liver Transplantation, *Scand J Gastroenterol*, **212**, 19–22.
32. Samuel, D. *et al.* (1995). Long-Term Clinical and Virological Outcome after Liver Transplantation for Cirrhosis Caused by Chronic Delta Hepatitis, *Hepatology*, **21**, 333–339.
33. Johnson, M.W. *et al.* (1996). Hepatitis C Viral Infection in Liver Transplantation, *Arch Surg*, **131**, 284–291.
34. Rosen, H.R. *et al.* (1996). Graft Loss Following Liver Transplantation in Patients with Chronic Hepatitis C, *Transplantation*, **62**, 1773–1776.
35. Russo, M.W. *et al.* (2004). Patient and Graft Survival in Hepatitis C Recipients after Adult Living Donor Liver Transplantation in the United States, *Liver Transpl*, **10**, 340–346.
36. Mulligan, D.C. and Klintmalm, G.B.G. (1995). Should Liver Transplantation Be Performed for Hepatitis B? *Clin Transplant*, **9**, 246–248.

37. Everhart, J.E. and Beresford, T.P. (1997). Liver Transplantation for Alcoholic Liver Disease: A Survey of Transplantation Programs in the United States, *Liver Transpl Surg*, **3**, 220–226.

38. Gane, E.J. *et al.* (1995). Ribavirin Therapy for Hepatitis C Infection Following Liver Transplantation, *Transplant Int*, **8**, 61–64.

39. Mazzaferro, V. *et al.* (1996). Liver Transplantation for the Treatment of Small Hepatocellular Carcinomas in Patients with Cirrhosis, *New Engl J Med*, **334**, 693–699.

40. Busuttil, R.W. *et al.* (1994). One Thousand Liver Transplants: The Lessons Learned, *Ann Surg*, **219**, 490–499.

41. Boillot, O. *et al.* (1995). Effects of Early Interferon Alfa Therapy for Hepatitis C Virus Infection Recurrence after Liver Transplantation, *Transplant Proc*, **27**, 2501.

42. Poves, I. *et al.* (1995). TIPSS: A Measure to Control Variceal Bleeding before Liver Transplantation, *Transplant Proc*, **27**, 2315–2316.

43. Menegaux, F. *et al.* (1994). Impact of Transjugular Intrahepatic Portosystemic Shunt on Orthotopic Liver Transplantation, *World J Surg*, **18**, 866–871.

44. Wood, R.P. *et al.* (1994). Liver Transplantation: The Last Ten Years, *Surg Clin North Am*, **74**, 1133–1154.

45. Castells, L. *et al.* (2007). Liver Transplant in HIV-HCV Coinfected Patients: A Case Control Study, *Transplantation*, **83**, 354–358.

46. Roland, M.E. and Stock, P.G. (2006). Liver Transplantation in HIV-Infected Recipients, *Semin Liver Dis*, **26**, 273–284.

47. Sudan, D. *et al.* (2002). Radiochemotherapy and Transplantation Allows Long-Term Survival for Nonresectable Hilar Cholangiocarcinoma, *Am J Transplant*, **2**, 774–779.

48. O'Grady, J.G. *et al.* (1989). Early Indicators of Prognosis in Fulminant Hepatic Failure, *Gastroenterology*, **97**, 439–445.

49. Bernuau, J. *et al.* (1986). Multivariate Analysis of Prognostic Factors in Fulminant Hepatitis B, *Hepatology*, **6**, 648–651.

50. Malinchoc, M. *et al.* (2000). A Model to Predict Poor Survival in Patients Undergoing Transjugular Intrahepatic Portosystemic Shunts, *Hepatology*, **31**, 864–871.

51. Velidedeoglu, E. *et al.* (2002). The Outcome of Liver Grafts Procured from Hepatitis C Donors, *Transplantation*, **73**, 582–587.

52. Marroquin, C.E. *et al.* (2001). Transplantation of Hepatitis C-Positive Livers in Hepatitis C-Negative Patients is Equivalent to Transplanting Hepatitis C-Negative Livers, *Liver Transpl*, **7**, 762–768.

53. Pedotti, P. *et al.* (2004). A Comparative Prospective Study of Two Available Solutions for Kidney and Liver Transplantation, *Transplantation*, **77**, 1540–1545.

54. Adam, R. *et al.* (2000). Normalised Intrinsic Mortality Risk in Liver Transplantation: European Liver Transplant Registry Study, *Lancet*, **356**, 621–627.

55. Briceno, J. *et al.* (2002). Influence of Marginal Donors on Liver Preservation Injury, *Transplantation*, **74**, 522–526.

56. Piratvisuth, T. *et al.* (1995). Contribution of True Cold and Rewarming Ischemia Times to Factors Determining Outcome after Orthotopic Liver Transplantation, *Liver Transpl Surg*, **1**, 296–301.

57. D'Alessandro, A. *et al.* (1995). Successful Extrarenal Transplantation from Non-Heart-Beating Donors. *Transplantation*, **59**, 977–982.

58. Casavilla, A. *et al.* (1995). Experience with Liver and Kidney Allografts from Non-Heart-Beating Donors, *Transplant Proc*, **28**, 2898.

59. Simmons, R.L. *et al.* (1984). *Manual of Vascular Access, Organ Donation, and Transplantation*, Springer-Verlag, New York/Berlin/Heidelberg/Tokyo.

60. Imagawa, D. *et al.* (1996). Rapid En Bloc Technique for Pancreas–Liver Procurement, *Transplantation*, **61**, 1605–1609.

61. Rizzi, P.M. *et al.* (1994). Neoadjuvant Chemotherapy after Liver Transplantation for Hepatocellular Carcinoma, *Transplant Proc*, **26**, 3568–3569.

62. Fleitas, M.G. *et al.* (1994). Could the Piggyback Operation in Liver Transplantation Be Routinely Used? *Arch Surg*, **129**, 842–845.

63. Bismuth, H. and Houssin, D. (1984) Reduced-Size Orthotopic Liver Graft in Hepatic Transplantation in Children, *Surgery*, **95**, 367–370.

64. Pichlmayr, R. *et al.* (1988). Transplantation Einer Spenderleber auf Zwei Empfänger (Split-Liver Transplantation), *Langenbecks Arch Chir*, **373**, 127–130.

65. Broelsch, C.E. *et al.* (1990). Application of Reduced-Size Liver Transplantation as Split Grafts, Auxiliary Orthotopic Grafts, and Living-Related Segmental Transplants, *Ann Surg*, **212**, 368–377.

66. Broelsch, C.E. *et al.* (1994). Living Donor for Liver Transplantation, *Hepatology*, **20**, 49S–55S.

67. Kuo, P. *et al.* (1995). Orthotopic Liver Transplantation with Selective Use of Venovenous Bypass, *Am J Surg*, **170**, 671–675.

68. Salizzoni, M. *et al.* (1994). Piggyback Techniques versus Classical Technique in Orthotopic Liver Transplantation: A Review of 75 Cases, *Transplant Proc*, **26**, 3552–3553.

69. Strong, R.W. *et al.* (1990). Successful Liver Transplantation from a Living Donor to Her Son, *New Engl J Med*, **322(21)**, 1505–1507.

70. Pomfret, E.A. *et al.* (2001). Live Donor Adult Liver Transplantation Using Right Lobe Grafts: Donor Evaluation and Surgical Outcome, *Arch Surg*, **136**, 425–433.

71. Grewal, H.P. *et al.* (2001). Surgical Technique for Right Lobe Adult Living Donor Living Transplantation without Venovenous Bypass or Portocaval Shunting and with Duct-to-Duct Biliary Reconstruction, *Ann Surg*, **233**, 502–508.

72. Trotter, J.F. *et al.* (2006). Documented Deaths of Hepatic Lobe Donors for Living Donor Liver Transplantation, *Liver Transpl*, **12**, 1485–1488.

73. Renz, J.F. and Roberts, J.P. (2000). Long-Term Complications of Living Donor Liver Transplantation, *Liver Transpl*, **6**, S73–S76.
74. New York State Department of Health. (2002). *Liver Donation: New York State Committee on Quality Improvement in Living Liver Donation*. Available at: http://www.health.state.ny.us/nysdoh/liver_donation (accessed 7 August 2011).
75. Kam, I. *et al.* (1987). Evidence That Host Size Determines Liver Size: Studies in Dogs Receiving Orthotopic Liver Transplants, *Hepatology*, **7**, 362–366.
76. Dahm, F., Georgiev, P. and Clavien, P.A. (2005). Small-for-Size Syndrome after Partial Liver Transplantation: Definition, Mechanisms of Disease and Clinical Implications, *Am J Transplant*, **5**, 2605–2610.
77. Trotter, J.F. *et al.* (2002). Adult-to-Adult Transplantation of the Right Hepatic Lobe from a Living Donor, *New Engl J Med*, **346**, 1074–1082.
78. Heffron, T.G. *et al.* (2002). Liver Transplant Induction Trial of Daclizumab to Spare Calcineurin Inhibition, *Transplant Proc*, **34**, 1514–1515.
79. Pageaux, G.P. *et al.* (French CHI-F-01 Study Group) (2004). Steroid Withdrawal at Day 14 after Liver Transplantation: A Double-Blind, Placebo-Controlled Study, *Liver Transpl*, **10**, 1454–1460.
80. Ringe, B. *et al.* (2001). A Novel Management Strategy of Steroid-Free Immunosuppression after Liver Transplantation: Efficacy and Safety of Tacrolimus and Mycophenolate Mofetil, *Transplantation*, **71**, 508–515.
81. Zavaglia, C. *et al.* (2005). Predictors of Long-Term Survival after Liver Transplantation for Hepatocellular Carcinoma, *Am J Gastroenterol*, **100**, 2708–2716.
82. Roayaie, S. *et al.* (2004). Recurrence of Hepatocellular Carcinoma after Liver Transplant: Patterns and Prognosis, *Liver Transpl*, **10**, 534–540.
83. Jacob, D.A. *et al.* (2006). Long-Term Follow-Up after Recurrence of Primary Biliary Cirrhosis after Liver Transplantation in 100 Patients, *Clin Transplant*, **20**, 211–220.
84. Gautam, M., Cheruvattath, R. and Balan, V. (2006). Recurrence of Autoimmune Liver Disease after Liver Transplantation: A Systematic Review, *Liver Transpl*, **12**, 1813–1824.
85. Verdonk, R.C. *et al.* (2006). Biliary Complications after Liver Transplantation: A Review, *Scand J Gastroenterol Suppl*, **243**, 89–101.
86. Noack, K. *et al.* (1993). The Greater Vulnerability of Bile Duct Cells to Reoxygenation Injury than to Anoxia: Implications for the Pathogenesis of Biliary Strictures after Liver Transplantation, *Transplantation*, **56**, 495–500.
87. Morelli, J. *et al.* (2001). Endoscopic Treatment of Post-Liver Transplantation Biliary Leaks with Stent Placement Across the Leak Site, *Gastrointest Endosc*, **54**, 471–475.
88. Saab, S. *et al.* (2000). Endoscopic Management of Biliary Leaks after T-tube Removal in Liver Transplant Recipients: Nasobiliary Drainage versus Biliary Stenting, *Liver Transpl*, **6**, 627–632.

89. Verdonk, R.C. *et al.* (2006). Anastomotic Biliary Strictures after Liver Transplantation: Causes and Consequences, *Liver Transpl*, **12**, 726–735.

90. Buis, C.I. *et al.* (2007). Nonanastomotic Biliary Strictures after Liver Transplantation, Part 1: Radiological Features and Risk Factors for Early vs. Late Presentation, *Liver Transpl*, **13**, 708–718.

91. Buis, C.I. *et al.* (2006). Causes and Consequences of Ischemic-Type Biliary Lesions after Liver Transplantation, *J Hepatobiliary Pancreat Surg*, **13**, 517–524.

92. Guichelaar, M.M. *et al.* (2003). Risk Factors for and Clinical Course of Nonanastomotic Biliary Strictures after Liver Transplantation, *Am J Transplant*, **3**, 885–890.

93. Verdonk, R.C. *et al.* (2007). Nonanastomotic Biliary Strictures after Liver Transplantation, Part 2: Management, Outcome, and Risk Factors for Disease Progression, *Liver Transpl*, **13**, 725–732.

94. Vallejo, G.H., Romero, C.J. and Vincente, J.C. (2005). Incidence and Risk Factors for Cancer after Liver Transplantation, *Crit Rev Oncol Hematol*, **56**, 87–99.

95. Takaki, A. *et al.* (2007). Short-Term High-Dose Followed by Long-Term Low-Dose Hepatitis B Immunoglobulin and Lamivudine Therapy Prevented Recurrent Hepatitis B after Liver Transplantation, *Transplantation*, **83**, 231–233.

96. Boillot, O. *et al.* (2003). Initial French Experience in Adult-to-Adult Living Donor Liver Transplantation, *Transplant Proc*, **35**, 962–963.

97. Foster, R., Zimmerman, M. and Trotter, J.F. (2007). Expanding Donor Options: Marginal, Living and Split Liver Donors, *Clin Liver Dis*, **11**, 417–429.

98. Olthoff, K.M. *et al.* (2005). Outcomes of 385 Adult-to-Adult Living Donor Liver Transplant Recipients: A Report from the A2 All Consortium, *Ann Surg*, **242**, 314–323.

99. Patel, S. *et al.* (2007). Living Donor Liver Transplantation in the United States: Identifying Donors at Risk for Perioperative Complications, *Am J Transplant*, **7**, 2344–2349.

100. Sarasin, F.P. *et al.* (2001). Living Donor Liver Transplantation for Early Hepatocarcinoma: A Life Expectancy and Cost-Effectiveness Perspective, *Hepatology*, **33**, 1073–1079.

101. Todo, S., Furukawa, H. and Japanese Study Group on Organ Transplantation. (2004). Living Donor Liver Transplantation for Adult Patients with Hepatocellular Carcinoma: Experience in Japan, *Ann Surg*, **240**, 451–459.

102. Tanaka, K. and Yamada, T. (2005). Living Donor Liver Transplantation in Japan and Kyoto University: What Can We Learn? *J Hepatol*, **42**, 25–28.

103. Middleton, P.F. *et al.* (2006). Living Donor Liver Transplantation — Adult Donor Outcomes: A Systematic Review, *Liver Transpl*, **12**, 24–30.

104. Trotter, J.F. *et al.* (2006). Documented Deaths of Hepatic Lobe Donors for Living Donor Liver Transplantation, *Liver Transpl,* **12**, 1485–1488.

105. Morioka, D. *et al.* (2007). Outcomes of Adult-to-Adult Living Donor Liver Transplantation: A Single Institution's Experience with 335 Consecutive Cases, *Ann Surg*, **245**, 315–325.
106. Ghobrial, R.M. *et al.* (2008). Donor Morbidity after Living Donation for Liver Transplantation, *Gastroenterology*, **135**, 468–476.
107. Karam, V.H. *et al.* (2003). Quality of Life in Adult Survivors Beyond 10 Years after Liver, Kidney, and Heart Transplantation, *Transplantation*, **76**, 1699–1704.
108. Tome, S. *et al.* (2008). Quality of Life after Liver Transplantation: A Systematic Review, *J Hepatol*, **48**, 567–577.

8

Heart Transplantation

Varun R. Kshettry and Vibhu R. Kshettry

8.1 History

Heart transplantation has evolved through extensive experimental development in surgical techniques, cardiopulmonary bypass, harvesting, and immunosuppression.[1] Alex Carrel and Charles Guthrie were the first to perform an experimental transplant at the University of Chicago in 1905, when they transplanted the heart of a puppy to the neck of an adult dog.[2,3] An hour after the operation, effective ventricular contraction occurred at a rate of 88 beats per minute for 2 hours. Nearly three decades after the Carrel experiment, Frank C. Mann at the Mayo Clinic in 1933 published the first methodical study of experimental heart transplantation.[4] He created a denervated heart model, transplanting a canine heart into the carotid-jugular circulation. Mann's heart model was the first to study the physiology of the transplanted organ and to describe the pathological changes of rejection.

Early experiments in orthotopic heart-lung transplantation were primarily centered on creating a simplified surgical technique and improving preservation of the graft and the recipient. To simplify the surgical technique, most of these initial attempts at heart transplant were combined heart-lung transplants to avoid multiple pulmonary venous anastomoses. Petrovich Demikhov, a Russian surgeon, was the first to report a successful heart-lung transplant in canines in 1951.[5] Lower and Shumway at Stanford University in 1960 reported the first successful series of prolonged survival — from 6 to 21 days — in dogs, with a simplified orthotopic heart transplant surgical technique.[6]

The first successful human heart transplantation was performed on December 3, 1967, by Christian Barnard in South Africa.[7] The recipient survived for 18 days, then died of pneumonia. Norman Shumway did the first successful heart transplant in the US on January 6, 1968.[8] These initial successes were followed by an exponential increase in the number of heart transplants. But enthusiasm decreased in the 1970s due to problems with rejection and other complications. It was not until cyclosporine was clinically introduced in the early 1980s that heart transplantation became common practice. Today, more than 250 centers worldwide perform heart transplants.

8.2 Indications

Heart transplant candidates require an aggressive and thorough screening process. As adult cardiac transplantation has progressed, recipient selection has been refined to balance the option to offer transplantation to sicker, complicated patients with recognition that this modality is a resource based on a severely limited donor pool. Generally, the indications for heart transplantation are end-stage heart failure (New York Heart Association (NYHA) class III or IV symptoms and failure of maximal medical therapy) with a poor long-term prognosis. About 40% of class IV heart failure die within one year in spite of optimal medical therapy.[9] End-stage heart disease typically includes an array of cardiomyopathies, most commonly ischemic or idiopathic dilated disease. The end-stage heart disease is not amenable to other medical or surgical therapy.

The pre-transplant workup includes cardiac catheterization with endomyocardial biopsy to rule out potentially treatable conditions, such as sarcoidosis or myocarditis. Candidates need to have no other organ dysfunction (apart from their heart) and be emotionally stable and compliant with medical advice and therapy with a good family support system.

Oxygen consumption, measured during maximal exercise, is used to objectively assess the candidate's capacity and cardiovascular reserve.

Candidates with peak oxygen consumption equal to, or less than, 10 ml/kg/min have poor one-year survival prospects, and so are listed for a transplant. However, those with peak oxygen consumption greater than 14 ml/kg/min have a 94% one-year chance of survival; they should defer the transplant unless they have other significant clinical concerns.[10] Left ventricular function is also a useful predictor of long-term survival. Patients with a left ventricular ejection fraction less than 20% have a one-year survival rate less than 50%. The current indications for placing candidates on the waiting list are listed below:

1. Cardiogenic shock or low output state with reversible end-organ dysfunction requiring mechanical support.
2. Low output state or refractory heart failure requiring continuous inotropic support.
3. Advanced heart failure signs and symptoms (NYHA Class III or IV) with objective documentation (generally via decrease in peak oxygen consumption on cardiopulmonary exercise testing) of marked functional limitation and poor one-year prognosis despite maximal medical therapy.
4. Recurrent or rapidly progressive heart failure symptoms unresponsive to maximized vasodilators and a flexible diuretic program.
5. Severe hypertrophic or restrictive cardiomyopathy with NYHA Class IV heart failure or anginal symptoms.

The many significant contraindications to a heart transplant are listed below:

1. Active infection.
2. Recent malignancy.
3. Pulmonary hypertension with irreversibly high pulmonary vascular resistance (greater than 6 Wood units during a vasodilator trial).
4. Diabetes mellitus and evidence of significant retinopathy, neuropathy, or nephropathy.
5. Myocardial infiltrative or inflammatory disease.
6. Active peptic ulcer disease.
7. Any systemic illness that would limit life expectancy or compromise functional rehabilitation.
8. Significant severe pulmonary parenchymal disease.
9. Irreversible renal dysfunction.
10. Severe peripheral vascular or cerebrovascular disease.

11. Irreversible hepatic dysfunction or cirrhosis.
12. Documented medical noncompliance.
13. Active substance abuse (including tobacco).
14. Untreated psychiatric illness.

Irreversible pulmonary, hepatic, or renal disease is considered contraindication; such disease markedly limits rehabilitation potential post transplant. Some degree of pre-transplant organ dysfunction is expected due to severe heart failure, but should not be present in the absence of a low output syndrome. Elevated pulmonary vascular resistance is a primary exclusionary criterion for a heart-lung transplant.[11] All heart transplant candidates need a complete psychosocial evaluation to identify potential social and behavioral problems that may require intervention pre or post transplant.

Age limits for heart transplantation are controversial. In the past, it was generally accepted that heart transplant recipients should be under age 50. Several transplant centers, however, have done heart transplants for patients in their 50s and 60s with good long-term results. Currently, patients less than 65 years of age are considered for transplant.

Indications for heart transplantation are similar in several respects for children, compared with adults. A transplant is indicated for any child with end-stage heart disease whose condition is refractory to maximal medical therapy or other surgical intervention. Cardiomyopathy and complex congenital heart disease — with or without myocardial failure — are the two main diagnostic groups. With children who have dilated cardiomyopathy or heart failure, no reliable predictors for poor survival are known. Deciding when to place them on the waiting list, if at all, is difficult.[12,13] General clinical indications include increasing heart failure despite maximal medical therapy. Some children are referred because of a congenital heart abnormality, before severe heart failure develops, when the natural history of the abnormality precludes long-term survival. Those with growth failure or cardiac cachexia should also be considered for a transplant. Importantly, children need a reliable caregiver to administrate immunosuppression and other post-transplant care.

Retransplantation remains controversial. A certain number of recipients will suffer progressive graft dysfunction. Despite maximal care after a heart transplant, chronic rejection and allograft coronary artery disease are major factors affecting long-term survival. Retransplantation in this sub-group has short-term survival similar to initial transplantation in critically ill patients. Additionally, limited donor organ availability and restrained financial resources complicate the issue of retransplantation.

8.3 Surgical Technique

8.3.1 Donor

Heart procurement is a routine part of a multiple-organ retrieval operation. The chest is opened through a midline sternotomy incision. The pericardium is opened and attached to the edges of the sternotomy with sutures. The heart is carefully inspected. Any evidence of myocardial contusion or other injury is noted. The overall contractility of the left and right ventricles is observed. The coronary arteries are palpated for coronary artery disease. If the heart is suitable for donation, further preparation for excision is carried out.

The superior and inferior vena cavae and ascending aorta are all encir-cled with tapes. A purse-string suture is placed in the ascending aorta for insertion of a cardioplegia cannula. When the abdominal viscera are mobilized and readied for removal, retrieval of the heart can proceed, Intravenous heparin (400 units/kg of body weight) is given. All central lines are removed. Removal of the heart begins with ligation and divi-sion of the superior vena cava. The inferior vena cava is partially divided to empty the heart of blood. The aorta is crossclamped at the base of the innominate artery. Then, 1000 cc of cold hyperkalaemic crystalloid car-dioplegic solution is infused into the aorta in order to achieve rapid car-diac arrest and protect the myocardium from ischemic injury. The heart is topically cooled with 4°C normal saline as an adjunct to cardiople-gia. After cardioplegia is completed, excision of the heart is begun. The inferior vena cava is divided flush with the right atrium. The heart is retracted to the right. The left pulmonary veins are divided close to the pericardium. Similarly, the right pulmonary veins are divided. Next, the distal main pulmonary artery and distal ascending aorta are divided. The heart is then removed, placed in cold saline, and packaged for the recipient hospital.

8.3.2 Recipient

After the arrival time of the donor heart is estimated and co-ordinated, the recipient is prepared for surgery. The chest is opened through a midline sternotomy incision. After heparinization, cardiopulmonary bypass is initiated via cannulas inserted in the ascending aorta at the level of the innominate artery, into the superior and inferior vena cavae. Both vena cavae are encircled with tapes and snared over the cannulas to establish total cardiopulmonary bypass. The body is systemically cooled to 28°C to prevent early rewarming of the donor heart.

The aorta is cross-clamped just proximal to the aortic cannula. The right atrium is transected, beginning midway between the tip of the right atrial appendage and the junction of the superior vena cava and the right atrium. This incision is carried inferiorly to the coronary sinus, leaving an adequate cuff of the right atrium anterior to the venous cannulas. Care is taken to avoid injuring the Swan–Ganz catheter, if present. Superiorly, the incision is carried to the root of the aorta. The left atrium is incised just posterior to the aorta. The aorta and pulmonary artery are transected at the level of the commissures of the valves. With both atria open, the right atrial septum is divided well anteriorly. The incisions in the septum and the lateral atrial wall join at the ostium of the coronary sinus. The cardiectomy is completed by an incision along the atrioventricular groove on the left side, leaving a cuff of left atrium around the pulmonary veins.

The donor heart is brought into the operating field. The left atrial cuff is fashioned by connecting pulmonary vein orifices with the incision. An oblique incision in the right atrial wall, from the inferior vena cava to the appendage, is made to match the recipient right atrium. When making this incision, injury to the sinoatrial node must be avoided. The atrial septum is carefully checked for patent foramen ovale. If present, it is repaired before the heart is implanted.

The pericardial cavity is irrigated with cold saline solution. The donor and recipient left atria are aligned and anastomosed with a running 3-0 polypropylene suture. The Swan–Ganz catheter, if present, is repositioned into the pulmonary artery. The two right atria are then anastomosed with a running 3-0 polypropylene suture. The donor and recipient pulmonary arteries are trimmed to size and anastomosed end to end with a running 4-0 polypropylene suture. The donor and recipient aorta are similarly trimmed and anastomosed end to end with a running two-layer 4-0 polypropylene suture. The patient's body is rewarmed. A vent site to remove air from the heart is placed in the ascending aorta. The cross-clamp is removed to restore perfusion to the heart. When heart function is satisfactory, the patient is weaned from cardiopulmonary bypass, heparin is reversed with protamine infusion, and the cannulas from the heart are removed. Once hemostasis is secured, the sternum is closed with drainage tubes in place.

The Lower and Shumway technique, as described above, has been the gold standard for many years.[14] Recently, many transplant centers are adopting a bicaval anastomoses technique in an attempt to preserve atrial contractility, sinus node function, and atrioventricular valve competence. These alternative surgical techniques sometimes have induced significant stenoses of the vena cavae anastomoses and to avoid these, modifications have been described by leaving a trapezoidal strip of the posterior wall of the right atrium as a connection between the superior vena cava, left atrium and inferior vena cava.[15]

8.4 Post–Operative Care

8.4.1 Intensive care unit

Recipients are taken to the intensive care unit for monitoring immediately after surgery. Strict attention to fluid management is maintained. Fluid overload and renal impairment are common after cardiopulmonary bypass and cyclosporine therapy. Diuresis is achieved with diuretics and low-dose dopamine. Recipients are also maintained on intravenous isoproterenol, for two to three days, due to its beneficial chronotropic effects and its ability to reduce pulmonary vascular resistance. Cardiovascular performance is optimized to improve oxygen delivery. Early ventilator weaning, based on physiologic respiratory parameters, is encouraged.

8.4.2 Immunosuppression

Improvements in immunosuppression and post-transplant care have largely been responsible for the tremendous success — in both short- and long-term survival rates — of heart transplantation. Rejection is one of the leading causes of death in the first post-transplant year.[16,17] Immunosuppression regimens are generally classified as either induction, maintenance, or rejection regimens.[18] Induction therapy is intense perioperative immunosuppressive therapy. Although it was originally designed to induce tolerance to the graft, this goal has not been realized. The benefit of induction therapy is a marked reduction in rejection in the early postoperative period. However, there is increased late rejection after induction therapy. Maintenance therapy generally consists of a combination of an antimetabolite (azathioprine or mycophenolate mofetil), a calcineurin inhibitor (cyclosporine or tacrolimus), and steroids. Maintenance regimens are evolving with efforts to diminish the nephrotoxicity of calcineurin inhibitors and metabolic toxicity of steroids. Combination therapy targets several distinct steps in T-cell activation and is thus designed to limit the toxicity of any one drug by allowing lower doses of several drugs. Specific maintenance regimens vary at different transplant centers and are based on age, presensitization, race, and previous rejection. These factors determine a patient's risk for rejection. Our current immunosuppressive protocol at the Minneapolis Heart Institute using a combination of triple drug therapy is outlined in Table 8.1.

8.4.3 Complications

Most deaths in the first post-transplant year are caused by acute rejection or infection. The development of these two problems is interrelated: Insufficient immunosuppression may lead to acute rejection, whereas over-immunosuppresion may result in opportunistic infections. Other complications include graft coronary artery disease, malignancy, and toxicity related to long-term drug therapy.

Rejection has been classified into cell mediated (most common) and antibody mediated (also known as humoral or vascular). Chronic rejection has been renamed "allograft coronary artery disease," since it is actually a type of vasculopathy. Factors associated with an increased risk of rejection include human leukocyte (HLA) mismatches,[19] female gender and younger donor hearts,[20,21] non-O blood type,[22] panel reactive antibody screen greater than 10%,[23,24] positive donor-specific crossmatch,[22] OKT3 murine monoclonal antibody sensitization,[24] cytomegalovirus infection,[25] and anti-HLA

Table 8.1 Immunosuppressive protocol for heart transplants.

	Pre-Op	Intra-Op	Post-Op	Maintenance	Rejection *ISHLT Grade		
					Mild IA or IB	Moderate 3A	Severe ≥3B
METHYLPREDNI-SOLONE		500 mg IV after coming off car-diopul-monary bypass	125 mg IV q12h ×3 doses			500 mg IV ×3 days Repeat biopsy within 1 week	500 mg IV ×3 days or antilymphocyte preparation Repeat biopsy within 1 week
CYCLOSPORINE	3 mg/kg p.o.		3–5 mg/kg/d increasing pending HPLC whole blood levels (ng/mL)	Trough levels: (0–3 mo: 175–225 4–6 mo: 125–175 6–12 mo: 100–150 >12 mo: 75–125	No change	No change No change	No change

(Continued)

Table 8.1 (*Continued*)

	Pre-Op	Intra-Op	Post-Op	Maintenance	Rejection *ISHLT Grade		
					Mild IA or IB	Moderate 3A	Severe ≥3B
TACROLIMUS	0.1 mg/kg p.o.		0.05–0.2 mg/kg/d Adjust pending tacrolimus level	0–1 mo: 10–20 ng/mL 1–3 mo: 10–15 ng/mL >3 mo: 5–10 ng/mL	No change	No change	No change
MYCO-PHENOLATE MOFETIL	1 gm p.o.		1–3 gm/day	1–3 gm/day	No change	No change	No change
AZATHIOPRINE			2–3 mg/kg/d p.o. Hold for WBC <3000/mm (check with MD)	2 mg/kg/d Taper to maintain WBC 4,000–6,000	No change	No change	No change
PREDNISONE			1.5 mg/kg/d Taper by 10 mg/day to maintenance	0.5 mg/kg/d for 1 month, then taper to 0.2 mg/kg/d over 6 months	No change	If no IV bolus recycle to 1.5 mg/kg/d and taper	Recycle after IV bolus or after OKT2

(Continued

Table 8.1 (*Continued*).

	Pre-Op	Intra-Op	Post-Op	Maintenance	Rejection *ISHLT Grade		
					Mild IA or IB	Moderate 3A	Severe ≥3B
DACLIZUMAB (Zenapax)			1 mg/kg ×5 doses First dose within 24 hours of transplant with subsequent doses q2wks ×4 Used in selected patients			Repeat biopsy at end of course	

*ISHLT Grade 2 rejection is considered borderline, and treatment is determined based on patient rejection history/clinical status.

antibodies.[26] Large multicenter trials have identified female gender, HLA mismatches, and the use of female or younger donors as the highest risk factors for rejection.[27]

Acute rejection is diagnosed by endomyocardial biopsy, the most useful and accurate method. Other noninvasive methods for detecting rejection have been proposed, but none are as useful. Endomyocardial biopsy is most commonly done by percutaneous access to the internal jugular vein, with biopsy forceps used to obtain pieces of tissue from the right ventricular septum — a technique developed by Caves, Billingham, and others.[28] This technique is associated with a false-negative rate of 2–4%,[27] so continual surveillance and re-evaluation are required. Cardiac biopsies are routinely obtained at weekly intervals in the early post-transplant period, then every three to six months for the first year, and then yearly. Biopsies are also routinely done after treatment of acute rejection episodes to ensure resolution or improvement. Endomyocardial biopsy specimens undergo grading according to guidelines established by the International Society of Heart Transplantation.[29]

Acute rejection is treated by augmenting immunosuppression, usually as a three-day pulse of intravenous steroids, followed by an oral taper. Resistant rejection is treated by antilymphocyte agents such as OKT3. Rejection episodes refractory to the above measures may be treated with experimental modes of therapy, such as total lymphoid irradiation, photophoresis, or Cytoxan. Newer immunosuppressive agents are continually being developed and may offer an advantage over current conventional rejection therapy.

Allograft coronary artery disease was formerly referred to as chronic rejection, now recognized as a misnomer. Graft coronary artery disease may form quite rapidly post transplant, or it may progress more slowly. Its precise pathophysiology is unclear. It tends to affect the large epicardial coronary and smaller branch vessels in a diffuse fashion, rendering angioplasty or bypass surgery impossible. Graft atherosclerosis is a leading cause of death and complications after the first post-transplant year.[30] Since the transplanted heart is denervated, recipients do not develop angina and usually present with overt congestive heart failure or sudden death. To monitor graft atherosclerosis, recipients undergo annual cardiac catheterization. Developing strategies to prevent the graft coronary artery disease is one of the most important areas of research at many transplant centers.

Immunosuppressed heart recipients are predisposed to life-threatening infections from a wide variety of common opportunistic organisms such as cytomegalovirus (CMV) and pneumocystis carinii. Infection prophylaxis at our institution includes daily trimethoprim-sulfamethoxazole, acyclovir, and nystatin for three months post transplant. Recipients require aggressive evaluation and a high index of suspicion for the development of infection as well as aggressive surveillance of potential infections. Every attempt should be made to treat only identified infections and to avoid indiscriminate use of antibiotics, lest fungal or resistant bacterial overgrowth should develop.

Chronic immunosuppression is also associated with an increased risk of lymphoproliferative malignancy. Malignancy reportedly accounts for 5% of all deaths after heart transplantation,[31, 32] often associated with opportunistic infection with Epstein–Barr virus.[32,33] Lymphoma is the malignancy most often encountered. Retrospective analysis indicates that the overall degree of immunosuppression correlates with the risk of lymphoma.

8.5 Results of Heart Transplantation

According to the International Society for Heart and Lung Transplantation Registry report, a total of 70,201 heart transplants in 338 transplant centers were done worldwide as of June 30, 2004.[34] The number of annual heart transplants has plateaued, with donor availability being the limiting factor. Survival has improved in the past 20 years; in the most recent era (1999 to 2003) rates were 83% at 1 year and 78% at 3 years. Risk factors for one-year mortality include: a prior transplant, ventricular assistance or ventilator support pre transplant, very young (less than one year of age) or very old (greater than 65 years of age) recipient age, female gender (recipient or donor), underlying congenital heart disease, and use of older (greater than 55 years of age) donor. Allograft ischemic time continues to be a risk factor, adding about a 10% increase in mortality for every hour of donor organ ischemia. In addition, recipients at risk for primary cytomegalovirus infections (donor positive/recipient negative) have a 20% higher mortality rate in the first post-transplant year.

8.6 Future Directions

8.6.1 Mechanical heart replacement

As a treatment of terminal heart failure, transplants have been remarkably successful. However, many patients die while waiting for a suitable donor heart. Mechanical cardiac assistance technology has progressed dramatically. Reliable univentricular support can now be provided with minimal thromboembolic and infectious complications. Increasingly, implantable ventricular assist devices are being used as a bridge to transplantation for selected patients who would otherwise die waiting for a heart. Wearable battery-powered left ventricular assist devices are currently being proposed for long-term mechanical circulatory assistance — an appealing alternative. The HeartMate left ventricular assist device (TCI, Woburn, MA, USA) has already been successfully implanted in over 3,000 patients as a bridge to heart transplantation. Cardiac replacement with a total artificial as a bridge to transplantation has also been successfully performed in patients requiring bi-ventricular support.

In addition, long-term use of implantable left ventricular assist device for end-stage heart failure has been clinically evaluated resulting in a significant clinical survival benefit and improved quality of life. A left ventricular assist device currently is becoming an acceptable alternative therapy in selected patients who are not candidates for cardiac transplantation.[35] Total artificial hearts are currently undergoing evaluation as destination therapy in a select group of patients. The AbioCor mechanical heart provides permanent replacement of a failing heart for patients who are not transplant candidates. The initial clinical trials have shown promising results, but long-term results and regulatory approval are still awaited.[36]

8.6.2 Bio-technologies

Despite dramatic progress in the field of cardiac transplantation, donor heart shortage has prompted many investigators to research the therapeutic possibility of xenotransplantation.[37] The concept of transplanting hearts from animals into human is intriguing but raises many immunological and ethical barriers. Advances in molecular biology have led to greater understanding of factors that are involved in rejection and have allowed genetic manipulation of donor animals. This genetic engineering of pigs can make their hearts appear less "foreign" and thus less prone to rejection; someday pig hearts may serve as an acceptable alternative to donor human hearts.

One area of exciting progress in the field of heart transplantation is cellular transplant. The concept of isolating and transplanting cells has already been successfully employed in transplantation of bone marrow and hematopoietic stem cells and is now a standard therapy. However, there has been recent progress toward the application of cellular transplantation for disease of the heart. A significant constraint of cellular transplantation is that the transplanted cells may not assume anatomic localization that would allow optimum function.[37] Tissue engineering, using synthetic or biological polymers, is being developed to support the growth and differentiation of cells of interest. Experimental tissue engineering to date includes the generation of blood vessels, heart valves, and heart muscle. Organogenesis, another potential approach to transplantation, is based on the observation that primitive cells can develop into tissues that resemble normal tissues. Therefore, organogenesis provides the possibility that stem cells derived from an individual with organ failure may be used to generate a new organ. However, at the current time there remain significant challenges in creating an organ that is of adequate size and of appropriate vasculature.

References

1. Ventura, H.O. and Muhammed, K. (2001). Historical Perspectives on Cardiac Transplantation: The Past as Prologue to Challenges for the 21st Century. *Curr Opin Cardiol*, **16**, 118–123.
2. Carrel, A. and Guthrie, C.C. (1905). The Transplantation of Veins and Organs *Am Med*, **10**, 1101–1102.
3. Carrel, A. (1907). The Surgery of Blood Vessels. *Bull Johns Hopkins Hosp*, **18**, 18–28.
4. Mann, F.C. *et al.* (1933). Transplantation of the Intact Mammalian Heart. *Arch Surg*, **26**, 219–224.

5. Demikhov, V.P. (1962). *Experimental Transplantation of Vital Organs*, Consultants Bureau, New York.
6. Lower, R.R. and Shumway, N.E. (1960). Studies on Orthotopic Homotransplantation of the Canine Heart. *Surg Forum*, **11**, 18–19.
7. Barnard, C.N. *et al.* (1967). A Human Cardiac Transplant: An Interim Report of a Human Successful Operation Performed at Groote Schuur Hospital, Cape Town. *S Afr Med J*, **41**, 1271–1274.
8. Reitz, B.A. (1990). 'Heart and Lung Transplantation', in Baumgartner, W.A. *et al.* (eds.), *Heart and Heart-Lung Transplantation*, Saunders, Philadelphia, pp. 1–14.
9. Effects of Enalapril on Mortality in Severe Congestive Heart Failure. Results of the Cooperative North Scandinavian Enalapril Survival Study (CONSENSUS). The CONSENSUS Trial Study Group. (1987). *New Engl J Med*, **316**, 1429–1435.
10. Mancini, D.M. *et al.* (1991). Value of Peak Exercise Oxygen Consumption for Optimal Timing of Cardiac Transplantation in Ambulatory Patients with Heart Failure. *Circulation*, **83**, 778–786.
11. Griepp, R.B. *et al.* (1971). Determinants of Operative Risk in Human Heart Transplantation. *Am J Surg*, **122**, 192–197.
12. Lewis, A.B. *et al.* (1991). Outcome of Infants and Children with Dilated Cardiomyopathy. *Am J Cardiol*, **68**, 365–369.
13. Addonizio, L.J. (1992). Cardiac Transplantation for Cardiomyopathies of Childhood. *Prog Pediatr Cardiol*, **1**, 72–80.
14. Lower, R.R. *et al.* (1961). Homovital Transplantation of the Heart. *J Thorac Cardiovasc Surg*, **41**, 196–201.
15. Tsilimingas, N.B. (2003). Modification of Bicaval Anastomosis: An Alternative Technique for Orthotopic Cardiac Transplantation. *Ann Thor Surg* **75**, 1333–1334.
16. Kirklin, J.K. *et al.* (1988). Analysis of Morbid Events and Risk Factors for Death after Cardiac Transplantation. *J Am Coll Cardiol*, **11**, 917–924.
17. Hosenpud, J.D. *et al.* (1995). The Registry of the International Society for Heart and Lung Transplantation: Twelfth Official Report. *J Heart Lung Transplant*, **14**, 805–815.
18. Lindenfeld, J. *et al.* (2004). Drug Therapy in the Heart Transplant Recipient Part I: Cardiac Rejection and Immunosuppressive Drugs. *Circulation*, **110**, 3734–3740.
19. Constanzo-Nordin, M.R. (1992). Cardiac Allograft Vasculopathy: Relationship with Acute Cellular Rejection and Histocompatibility. *J Heart Lung Transplant*, **11**, S90–103.
20. Crandall, B.G. *et al.* (1988). Increased Cardiac Allograft Rejection in Female Heart Transplant Recipients. *J Heart Lung Transplant*, **7**, 419–423.
21. Renlund, D.G. *et al.* (1987). Age-Associated Decline in Cardiac Allograft Rejection. *Am J Med*, **83**, 391–398.

22. Lavee, J. *et al.* (1991). Influence of Panel-Reactive Antibody and Lympho-cytotoxic Crossmatch on Survival after Heart Transplantation. *J Heart Lung Transplant*, **10**, 921–930.

23. Kormos, R.L. *et al.* (1988). Immunologic and Blood Group Compatibility in Cardiac Transplantation. *Transplant Proc*, **20**, 741–742.

24. Hammond, E.H. *et al.* (1990). Relationship of OKT3 Sensitization and Vas-cular Rejection in Cardiac Transplant Patients Receiving OKT3 Rejection Prophylaxis. *Transplantation*, **50**, 776–782.

25. Normann, S.J. *et al.* (1991). Acute Vascular Rejection of the Coronary Arteries in Human Heart Transplantation: Pathology and Correlations with Immunosuppression and Cytomegalovirus Infection. *J Heart Lung Transplant*, **10**, 674–687.

26. Suciu-Foca, N. *et al.* (1991). The Role of Anti-HLA Antibodies in Heart Transplantation. *Transplantation*, **51**, 716–724.

27. Spiegelhalter, D.J. and Stovin, P.G.I. (1983). An Analysis of Repeated Biopsies Following Cardiac Transplantation. *Statis Med*, **2**, 33–40.

28. Caves, P.K. *et al.* (1973). Percutaneous Transvenous Endomyocardial Biopsy in Human Heart Recipients: Experience with a New Technique. *Ann Thor Surg*, **16**, 325–336.

29. Billingham, M.E. *et al.* (1990). A Working Formulation for the Standardiza-tion of Nomenclature in the Diagnosis of Heart and Lung Rejection: Heart Rejection Study Group. The International Society for Heart Transplantation. *J Heart Transplant*, **9**, 587–592.

30. Hunt, S.A. *et al.* (1994). In Hurst, J.W. *et al.* (eds.), *The Heart*, McGraw-Hill, New York, pp. 629–636.

31. Kriett, J.M. and Kaye, M.P. (1991). The Registry of the International Society for Heart and Lung Transplantation: Eighth Official Report. *J Heart Lung Transplant*, **10**, 491–498.

32. Young, L. *et al.* (1989). Expression of Epstein–Barr Virus Transformation-Associated Genes in Tissues of Patients with EBV Lymphoproliferative Disease. *New Engl J Med*, **321**, 1080–1085.

33. Hanto, D.W. *et al.* (1981). The Epstein–Barr Virus (EBV) in the Pathogenesis of Posttransplant Lymphoma. *Transplant Proc*, **13**, 756–760.

34. Taylor, D.O. *et al.* (2005). Registry of the International Society for Heart and Lung Transplantation: Twenty-Second Official Adult Heart Transplant Report. *J Heart Lung Transplant*, **24**, 945–955.

35. Rose, E.A. *et al.* (2001). Long-Term Use of a Left Ventricular Assist Device for End-Stage Heart Failure. *New Engl J Med*, **345**, 1435–1443.

36. Samuels, L.E. and Dowling, R. (2003). Total Artificial Heart: Destination Therapy. *Cardiol Clin*, **21**, 115–118.

37. Ogata, K. and Platt, J.L. (2004). Potential Applications and Prospects for Car-diac Xenotransplantation. *J Heart Lung Transplant*, **23**, 515–526.

9

Corneal Transplantation

Chad K. Rostron

There are estimated to be around 2,500 corneal grafts carried out per annum in the UK,[1] and five-year graft survival for patients having transplants for the corneal disease of keratoconus can be better than 95%.[2] However, in higher risk indications for keratoplasty such as re-grafts, five-year graft survival may be less than 50%.

The cornea can be divided into three functional layers: the external epithelium, the stroma (which forms the major bulk of the cornea), and the inner endothelial layer (Figure 9.1).

Each of these corneal layers can be transplanted in isolation, but most commonly the full thickness of the diseased cornea of the patient is exchanged for a similar piece of donor tissue in a penetrating keratoplasty. Usually only a central button of 7 to 8 mm diameter is excised with a circular trephine blade, and then sutured into a similar-sized hole cut in the recipient's cornea (Figure 9.2).

Initial attempts at penetrating keratoplasty with xenogenic material were unsuccessful, but Bigger achieved the first successful corneal homograft in his pet gazelle in 1835.[3] The first successful human corneal homograft to be carried out was attributed to Zirm in 1905.[4] The pioneers of keratoplasty were hampered by the lack of appropriate suture materials to secure the graft, and the slow wound healing of the corneal stroma, which lead to frequent complications and failure.

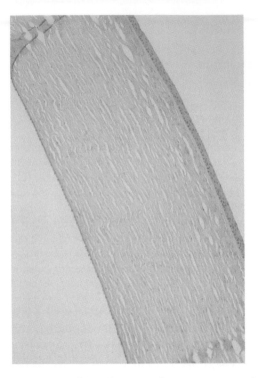

Figure 9.1 Transverse section through a normal cornea — central corneal thickness is around 530 microns.

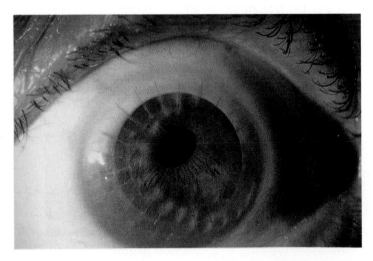

Figure 9.2 Clear 8.0 mm diameter penetrating corneal graft in a case of trachomatous corneal scarring. Multiple interrupted 11'0' polyester sutures *in situ*.

9.1 Corneal Structure and Function

The healthy cornea is smoothly curved, and transparent, and is the major refracting surface of the optical system of the eye. It also constitutes the anterior portion of the eyeball in continuity with the sclera, and acts as a physical barrier to the ingress of infection into the eye.

The near perfect transparency of the cornea to visible light is achieved because the tissue is avascular, and constituted of elements significantly smaller than the wavelength of light.[5] The bulk of the stroma is made of a regular lattice of collagen fibres in a glycosaminoglycan matrix, with occasional keratocytes scattered between the fibre bundles or lamellae (Figure 9.3). Nutrition for the keratocytes is supplied by aqueous humour diffusing from the anterior chamber into the stroma, but the regular spacing of the collagen fibres is maintained only by the cornea being kept in a state of relative dehydration. The inner endothelial layer continually pumps fluid out of the stroma back into the anterior chamber, whilst the epithelium forms an impermeable barrier to the influx of fluid from the tear film.

When these mechanisms break down, the cornea becomes oedematous, and the fluid lakes formed within the stroma cause loss of transparency due to light scatter. Although a corneal epithelial defect will allow fluid from the tear film to enter the stroma and cause oedema, the problem is generally

Figure 9.3 Transmission electron micrograph of corneal stroma showing regular lattice-like arrangement of collagen fibres.

short-lived, as the epithelium has considerable regenerative capacity and epithelial defects are rapidly covered by adjacent cells migrating. Endothelial defects, however, cause persistent corneal oedema as the endothelium has virtually no natural regenerative capacity.

9.2 Indications for Penetrating Keratoplasty

9.2.1 Endothelial failure

The corneal endothelium is a monolayer of cells with a density of over $3000/mm^2$ in infancy. Throughout life there is a progressive decline in cell density, and if the count falls below a level of around $500/mm^2$ there is irreversible corneal decompensation with oedema. This is termed 'bullous keratopathy', since fluid collects not just in the stroma but also between the epithelial cells, because only the cells in the outermost layer of the epithelium are linked by tight junctions. The intercellular fluid lakes form small bullae that cause the epithelial surface to become microscopically irregular like ground glass, thus further degrading the corneal transparency. If the epithelial bullae become large they may rupture and produce pain and lachrymation, and also open up a path for potential secondary infection of the cornea.

Primary endothelial failure is seen in Fuchs' corneal dystrophy — a pre-senile endothelial degeneration in which the endothelial cell layer becomes progressively depleted. Endothelial failure is also seen secondary to other factors such as intraocular inflammation or surgical trauma. With cataract surgery being carried out predominantly in the geriatric age group, it is not surprising that aphakic or pseudophakic bullous keratopathy are major indications for penetrating keratoplasty.

9.2.2 Keratoconus

Keratoconus is a corneal degeneration in which there is progressive thinning and ectasia of the central or para-central corneal stroma. The irregularity of corneal contour causes progressive visual distortion. The condition is genetically linked to a number of other syndromes including Down's, Ehlers–Danlos', Marfan's and atopy. Contact lenses are used to correct the vision in the earlier stages, but if it becomes more severe,

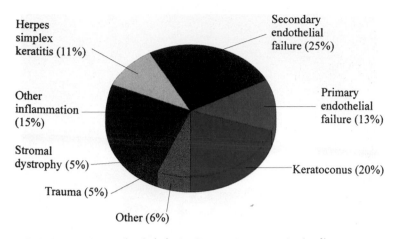

Figure 9.4 Proportions of ophthalmic diagnostic categories leading to penetrating keratoplasty (after Vail *et al.*[15]).

keratoplasty may be required. Keratoconus is currently the most frequent single indication for keratoplasty in the UK (Figure 9.4).

9.2.3 Infection and other indications

Worldwide, blindness from corneal disease ranks only second to blindness from cataract, and it is estimated that, of the many millions of people suffering from trachoma, some six million are blind.[6] The majority live in developing countries, where trachoma occurs through fly vector transmission in association with overcrowding and poor sanitation.

In the West, Herpes simplex has historically been a significant cause of corneal scarring, now less common since the introduction of effective topical antivirals (Figure 9.5). Corneal infections relating to contact lens wear are however increasing — pathogens such as Pseudomonas and Acanthamoeba can cause severe corneal ulceration and extensive tissue destruction.

9.3 Technique of Penetrating Keratoplasty

In endothelial failure, a large graft is needed to transplant sufficient donor endothelial cells to maintain the clarity of the whole cornea. Large grafts, however, have their edge close to the vascular limbus so it is more likely that the graft/host junction will become vascularised, increasing the risk of graft rejection. If there is a patient suffering from some form of stromal disease

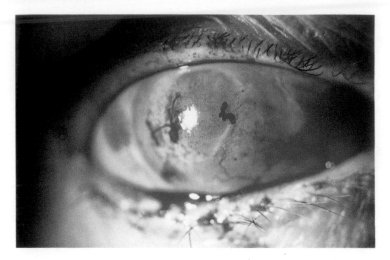

Figure 9.5 Recurrence of herpes simplex keratitis in a rejected corneal graft. The dendritic pattern of epithelial ulceration is highlighted by staining with Rose Bengal. Reactivation of herpes may be promoted by the use of the topical steroids which are required to suppress graft rejection.

only, then a small graft centred on the optical axis is sufficient to restore a clear visual pathway. However, a small graft has its suture line near to the visual axis, so the resulting local uneven corneal surface contour impairs the visual result obtained by creating astigmatism.

A major advance for keratoplasty has been the introduction of visco-elastic agents, such as sodium hyaluronate, which can be injected into the anterior chamber to cushion the graft and provide a protective barrier against trauma to the donor endothelium whilst the graft is being fixated. In addition, nylon mono-filament sutures have helped transform keratoplasty into the successful procedure that it is. Non-biodegradable polyester monofilament is being adopted by some surgeons now, since it can remain in the cornea without the need for removal.

9.4 Post–Operative Management

Corneal transplantation is blessed by the benefit of the opportunity for topical drug application, by which method one can achieve local tissue concentrations of drugs well in excess of those that would be tolerated with systemic administration. Typically, a keratoplasty patient will receive topical dexamethasone drops six times per day for a month, then four times per day for three months, gradually tapered off over the course of a year. However, long-term steroid administration can lead to cataract formation, and a proportion of patients respond idiosyncratically to topical steroids by developing secondary glaucoma. Both these iatrogenic complications can have a significant impact on the visual recovery of patients without, of course, being reflected in crude rates of graft survival.

Systemic steroids are generally reserved for high-risk patients with heavily vascularised corneas, or those undergoing re-grafts. Systemic immunosuppressants such as azathioprine and cyclosporine carry a greater risk of potentially fatal side effects, so some ophthalmologists feel that the use of such drugs cannot be justified in corneal transplantation, however severe the visual impairment.

9.5 Donor Tissue Selection and Preservation

Because the cell density and viability of donor endothelium can be assessed *in vitro*, the ophthalmic criteria for donor selection can be broad. The majority of retrieved donor eyes come from cadaveric donors, and even up to 48 hours post-mortem acceptable endothelial cell survival is sometimes found. The majority of UK and European eye banks use organ culture at 34°C to maintain the donor corneo-scleral segments. This method of preservation enables corneas to be kept readily for four to six weeks and so helps to regulate fluctuations of supply and demand, thus allowing keratoplasty to be carried out as a scheduled routine procedure.

In the UK, corneal donors are serologically screened for HIV, HBsAg, HCV, HTLV I & II, and syphilis, but not for CMV, as corneal recipients are rarely systemically immunosuppressed. The whole globe is enucleated and transported to the eye bank, where it is chemically disinfected, and a 17 mm diameter corneo-scleral segment excised (Figure 9.6).

At this stage a preliminary evaluation of the state of the endothelium is carried out after vital staining with Trypan blue (Figure 9.7). After a week in organ culture the medium is checked for bacterial and fungal contamination (Figure 9.8).

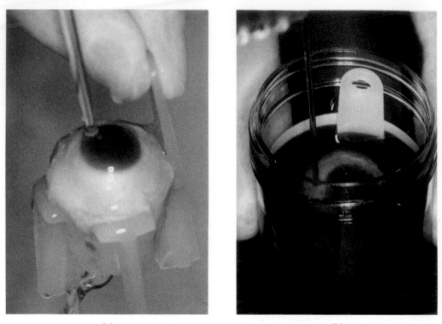

(a)   (b)

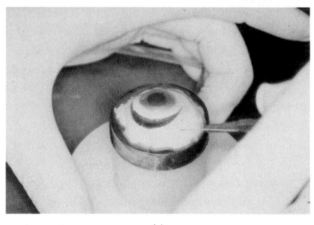

(c)

Figure 9.6 (a) Enucleated globes are washed copiously with sterile saline to remove surface contamination. (b) The globe is immersed in povidine iodine solution for further microbiological decontamination. (c) The corneo-scleral disc is excised from the globe.

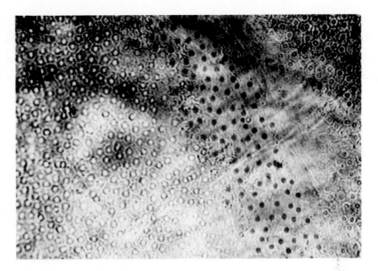

Figure 9.7 The endothelium is examined at 200 times magnification and the cell density determined. Dead or dying cells stain positively with Trypan blue.

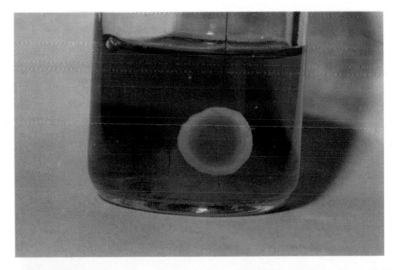

Figure 9.8 The corneo-scleral segment is suspended in organ culture fluid and maintained at 34°C for up to six weeks.

A few days before transplantation the tissue endothelium is reassessed, and the culture medium is changed to one containing high molecular weight dextran as an osmotic agent to dehydrate the donor tissue, which tends to become oedematous in the organ culture medium. The dextran solution is also checked for microbial contamination before transplantation.

9.6 Post-Operative Course of the Graft

During organ culture, the corneal epithelium becomes attenuated, and may slough off during surgery, or it may be intentionally removed to reduce the antigenic load, so that grafts may have a complete epithelial defect on the first post-operative day (Figure 9.9). Graft oedema at this stage is inevitable, with fluid ingress into the stroma both from the epithelial side and also from the endothelial side at the graft/host junction, and at any other areas of endothelial defect. Epithelial cover is usually re-established within a few days, but endothelial migration is considerably slower, and in all penetrating grafts the central endothelial cell count declines progressively over the first year or two by an order of around 50% as the endothelial cells migrate

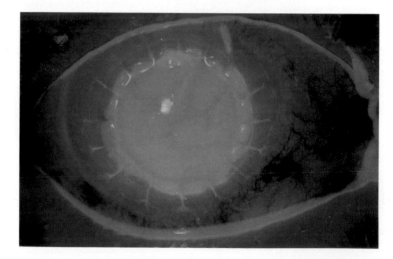

Figure 9.9 Corneal graft one day post-operatively showing a near total epithelial defect stained with fluorescein dye. There is early re-epithelialisation seen superiorly.

to cover areas of defect. For this reason a minimum donor endothelial cell density of 2000/mm^2 is considered mandatory if there is not to be an unacceptable rate of graft decompensation.

Grafts that are oedematous from day one, and fail to clear, are considered primary failures. With careful pre-operative assessment of donor tissue the rate of primary failures in penetrating keratoplasty is less than 1%. However, secondary endothelial failure is the commonest cause of late graft failure and is brought about by endothelial cell loss from trauma at the time of surgery, combined with progressive endothelial cell attrition from inflammation, age-related degeneration, drug toxicity and other unknown factors.

9.6.1 Graft rejection

Graft rejection is the major cause of graft failure, occurring particularly in the first year or two after grafting, but is sometimes seen after many years of successful tolerance of the donor tissue. Each of the three functional layers of the cornea can undergo rejection individually, and the characteristic clinical presentation of endothelial cell rejection was first described by Khodadoust in 1969 (Figure 9.10).[7] A linear front on the endothelium advances across

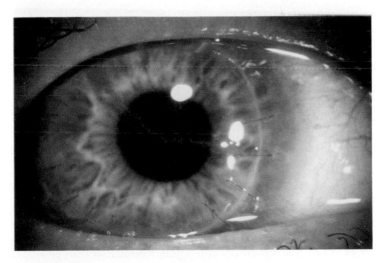

Figure 9.10 Penetrating corneal graft with epithelial rejection line running obliquely across the cornea.

the posterior surface of the graft, leaving behind damaged endothelium with overlying stromal and epithelial oedema. Epithelial rejection may follow a similar linear pattern, although it is rarely seen, as on all grafts the donated epithelium is progressively replaced by host cells, due to the natural centripetal migration of the epithelial cell sheet. Stromal rejection may be seen as fluffy white patches in the stroma. If patients are properly counselled to report immediately should they develop blurring of vision, photophobia, or ciliary congestion, then treatment of rejection can be commenced promptly, and the graft may be saved in the majority of cases. Treatment of rejection will consist typically of intensive topical steroids and mydriatics, with additional subconjunctival and systemic steroids.

Visual recovery after penetrating keratoplasty is generally slow. There is scanty re-innervation of the graft, and the epithelium on the graft may have a trophic disturbance (hurricane or vortex keratopathy). Uneven tension in the corneal sutures produces topographic distortion of the graft surface with regular and irregular astigmatism. This may not resolve until the sutures are removed, but with stromal wound healing being naturally slow, and inhibited by topical steroid application, elective suture removal cannot generally be carried out until at least one year post-operatively (Figure 9.11). Loose

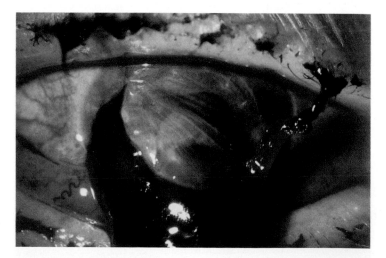

Figure 9.11 Traumatic rupture of corneal graft wound two years post-operatively with expulsive haemorrhage. Corneal wound healing is slow particularly when inhibited by topical steroids.

sutures, or suture removal, create local tissue disturbance and an inflammatory response in the cornea, which may precipitate graft rejection.

9.7 Tissue–Matched Corneal Grafting

One of the first studies to show the benefit of tissue matching in corneal transplantation was carried out by Batchelor and Casey in East Grinstead.[8] They studied HLA A and B types in a series of randomly allocated grafts, and found the best graft survival was in the group with the least mismatches. The effect was most marked in the high-risk group of patients who had corneal vascularisation or previous graft rejection, and in this group there was progressive reduction in graft survival with each increase in the number of A or B mismatches (Figure 9.12).

The study was carried out blind with random allocation of the corneas, so inevitably the number of patients in the well matched groups was small. Overall, one-year graft survival was only 33%, possibly indicating that this patient cohort was at particularly high risk in comparison to the condition of the average patient undergoing keratoplasty. Several other large studies from other centres have confirmed the benefit of matching HLA A and B.[9–11] However, a large multicentre study from the USA failed to demonstrate any benefit from HLA A and B matching. In comparison to Batchelor and Casey's study, three-year graft survival in the American study was 59%, indicating that the carefully controlled post-operative treatment regime may have been effective in masking any benefit from matching, and/or that the proportion of genuinely high risk cases was not so great.[12] More recent studies in Europe have again confirmed the benefits of Class I matching.[13,14]

There have also been a number of studies of the benefit of HLA DR matching. Some have shown positive benefit from matching; some have failed to show any effect. One study showed an increased risk of rejection with a good DR match.[15] All of these studies used serological methods for typing which have less specificity than in Class I typing, and are also particularly difficult for typing corneal donors when the viability of cadaveric donor leucocytes is often poor. A single study of Class II matching using genotyping by RFLP did show benefit in a high-risk group,[16] and a more recent study with Class II genotyping by PCR-SSP showed benefit of combined Class I and II matching in a normal risk group of patients.[14]

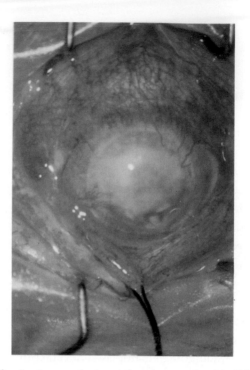

Figure 9.12 Graft rejection results in graft oedema and epithelial breakdown with the possibility of secondary bacterial ulceration. Chronic graft oedema leads to neovascularisation of the cornea and significantly reduces the chance of a further graft being successful, due to the vascularity of the bed and the prior sensitisation of the recipient to donor antigens.

9.8 Partial Thickness or Lamellar Keratoplasty

Partial thickness transplantation of individual corneal layers has the advantage of specifically targeting the diseased tissue layer or layers rather than replacing the full thickness of the cornea, when parts of the recipient cornea may still be healthy and possibly in a better condition than the donor tissue.

Thus where there is disease of the corneal stroma, but a functional corneal endothelium, then a partial thickness graft leaving the recipient endothelium *in situ* can remove the pathology without introducing the risk of endothelial rejection and associated graft failure (Figure 13(a) and (b)). Although an anterior lamellar graft may have its epithelium and stromal keratocytes rejected

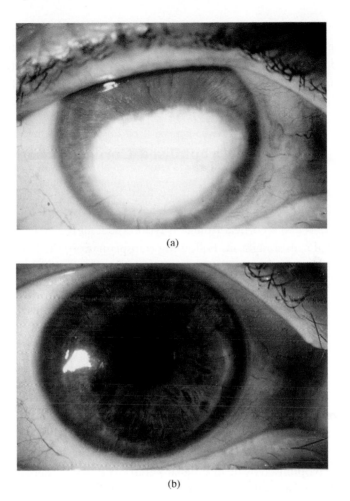

(a)

(b)

Figure 9.13 (a) Dense lipid infiltration of the cornea from neovascularisation of the stroma following herpes zoster ophthalmicus. (b) The same eye one year post-operatively following deep lamellar keratoplasty with lyophilised tissue.

by the host, this rarely leads to graft failure, as the host epithelium readily replaces any donor epithelial cells lost, and with time, host keratocytes can migrate into the donor stroma.

Despite these benefits, anterior lamellar keratoplasty currently only accounts for around 15% of corneal grafts performed in the UK, although the proportion of lamellar grafts is increasing. The procedure is more time-consuming and technically more difficult than penetrating keratoplasty, and the visual results may not always be perfect when the bed of the graft/host interface is irregular or undergoes fibrosis. However, improved instrumentation and microsurgical technique can now allow complete resection of the diseased stroma, leaving only the host Descemet's membrane and endothelium, with potentially excellent visual results.

9.9 Freeze-Dried or Lyophilised Corneal Tissue

Although fresh corneal tissue can be used for lamellar keratoplasty, the viability of the donor epithelium or keratocytes is not essential for the success of the graft. When a corneal lamella is lyophilised, all the cells in it die and the epithelial cells slough off. Following transplantation, the keratocyte cell debris is rapidly dispersed (Figure 9.14).

In an experimental model, a xenogenic lyophilised lamellar graft transplanted as an inter-lamellar inlay is not rejected. If a penetrating xenograft is then placed in the same recipient cornea, adjacent to the lyophilised lamella, it is rejected but the lyophilised tissue is unaffected.[17] Lyophilised corneal tissue not only fails to provoke rejection but also does not seem to sensitise the recipient to its donor antigens, presumably because the stimulus from the transplanted, but dead, keratocytes is too short-lived. Once lyophilised, a cornea can be preserved in a vacuum vial at room temperature for several months, and the convenience of this storage method made it popular for distribution of prelathed lenticules for epikeratophakia (Figure 9.15).

By using lyophilised tissue in lamellar keratoplasty when there is a possibility of the need for a subsequent penetrating graft, the risk of the eye being presensitised to donor antigens from the first lamellar graft is avoided. In addition, rejection of fresh lamellar grafts is usually associated with interface neo-vascularisation, which can impair corneal transparency, so the long-term visual outcome of rejection-free lyophilised tissue may prove to be advantageous over fresh tissue lamellar grafting.

9.10 Epithelial Transplantation

Occasionally there is failure of corneal epithelial regeneration due to epithelial stem cell depletion arising from, for instance, severe chemical

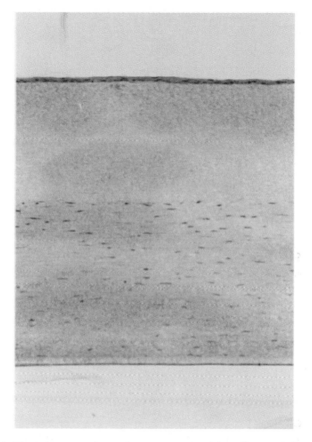

Figure 9.14 Transverse section of an experimental epikeratophakia graft in an animal model five days post-operatively. The recipient epithelium has just covered the graft, but as yet there is no repopulation of the lyophilised donor stroma. The donor keratocytes have dispersed and the donor stroma appears amorphous. The recipient stroma beneath has a normal keratocyte population.

injury to the anterior segment, or from autoimmune disease. Transplantation of epithelial sheets containing limbal stem cells can restore epithelial integrity in an eye otherwise doomed to progressive corneal scarring and melting from epithelial deficiency.[18] Autologous epithelial sheets grown from stem cells taken from the contralateral eye can be transplanted, but when this is not feasible then homologous transplantation can be carried out.[19] It seems likely that the fate of such grafts is short lived, but may be sufficient to stabilise an otherwise hopeless condition.

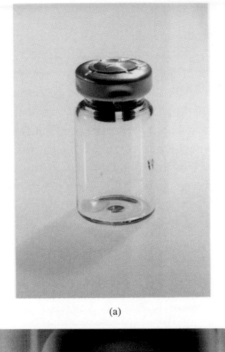

(a)

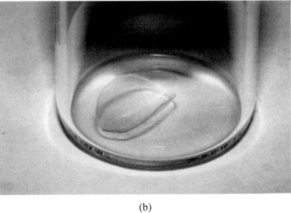

(b)

Figure 9.15 (a) Lyophilised corneal lenticule sealed under vacuum in a vial. These lenticules have a nominal shelf life of three months at room temperature. (b) Close-up view of corneal lenticule.

9.11 Endothelial Transplantation

After a hundred years of penetrating grafts, an amazing transformation in keratoplasty has recently been realised with the development of techniques of endothelial transplantation. Whilst the chance of obtaining corneal transparency following a penetrating keratoplasty is high, this unfortunately does not necessarily equate with restoration of good vision, since the shape of the cornea is critical to its powerful optical function, and even small degrees of deviation in its shape (by an order of microns) lead to visual distortion and image degradation. Even with the most careful suturing technique, there is virtually always residual optical error in a penetrating graft, with regular and irregular astigmatism, and this has been a perennial source of frustration for ophthalmic surgeons and their patients. However, by replacement of the endothelial layer alone, the patient's cornea can be left without disturbance of its external profile, and this allows rapid visual rehabilitation with an excellent optical outcome.

The first successful endothelial grafts involved transplantation of a thin sliver of posterior stroma together with the endothelium and Descemet's membrane, after removal of a similar slice of tissue from the recipient (deep lamellar endothelial keratoplasty: DLEK).[20] Since resection of these posterior layers from the patient's cornea is technically difficult, the surgical method rapidly evolved to one where only the Descemet's/endothelial complex was removed from the patient (Descemet's Stripping Endothelial Keratoplasty: DSEK). To facilitate preparation of the donor tissue layers, an alternative method to manual lamellar dissection uses a motorised microkeratome to slice the donor corneo–scleral segment while it is mounted on an artificial anterior chamber (Descemet's Stripping Automated Endothelial Keratoplasty: DSAEK). In both DSEK and DSAEK, although only Descemet's and the endothelium are removed from the recipient, the transplanted tissue has a thin posterior stromal lamella adherent to it, which makes handling of the tissue easier for the surgeon.

The most recent advance in endothelial grafting is to transplant only the Descemet's/endothelial complex (Descemet's Membrane Endothelial Keratoplasty: DMEK).[21] Once the Descemet's/endothelial sheet has been detached from the donor cornea it forms a slender scroll which can be injected through a 3.5 mm corneal incision into the patient's anterior chamber. The sheet must then be atraumatically unrolled and floated up onto the back of the patient's cornea on an air bubble, before becoming spontaneously adherent to the stroma.

Whilst all these techniques of endothelial transplantation can have excellent outcomes, there is an increased risk of failure from early graft dehiscence, or from damage to the endothelial cells during transplantation. However, continued advances in microsurgical technique have made these developments in keratoplasty a realistic option for many patients, and the improved quality, and speed, of visual rehabilitation make the additional technical complexity of the procedures well worthwhile. Corneal transplantation is already remarkably successful, and advances in the field continue to broaden the scope and benefits of the treatments available.

References

1. UKT (2007). *UK Transplant Activity Report 2006–2007*, 37–42. Available at: http://www.organdonation.nhs.uk/ukt/statistics/transplant_activity_report/ archive_activity_reports/pdf/ukt/transplant_activity_uk_2006-2007.pdf (accessed 2 April 2011).
2. Williams, K.A. *et al.* (1995). How Successful is Corneal Transplantation? A Report from the Australian Corneal Graft Register, *Eye*, **9**, 219–227.
3. Bigger, S.L. (1837). An Enquiry into the Possibility of Transplanting the Cornea, with the View of Relieving Blindness Caused by Several Diseases of that Structure. *J Med Soc Dublin*, **11**, 408–417.
4. Zirm, E. (1906). Eine erfolgreiche totale Keratoplastik. *Albrecht von Graefes Arch Ophthalmol*, **64**, 580–593.
5. Farrell, R.A. *et al.* (1973). Wave-Length Dependencies of Light Scattering in Normal and Cold Swollen Rabbit Corneas and their Structural Implications. *J Physiol*, **233**, 589–612.
6. Foster, A. and Johnson, G.J. (1990). Magnitude and Causes of Blindness in the Developing World. *Int Ophthalmol*, **14**, 135–140.
7. Khodadoust, A.A. and Silverstein, A.M. (1969). Transplantation and Rejection of Individual Cell Layers of the Cornea. *Invest Ophthalmol Vis Sci*, **8**, 180–195.
8. Batchelor, J.R. *et al.* (1976). HLA Matching and Corneal Grafting. *Lancet*, **1**, 551–554.
9. Sanfilippo, F. *et al.* (1986). Reduced Graft Rejection with Good HLA-A and B Matching in High-Risk Corneal Transplantation. *New Engl J Med*, **315**, 29–35.

10. Völker-Dieben, H.J. *et al.* (1987). Hierarchy of Prognostic Factors for Corneal Allograft Survival. *Aust NZ J Ophthalmol*, **15**, 11–18.
11. Boisjoly, H.M. *et al.* (1986). HLA-A, B and DR Matching in Corneal Transplantation. *Ophthalmology*, **93**, 1290–1297.
12. The Collaborative Corneal Transplantation Studies Research Group. (1992). The Collaborative Corneal Transplantation Studies (CCTS). Effectiveness of Histocompatibility Matching in High-Risk Corneal Transplantation. *Arch Ophthalmol*, **110**, 1392–1403.
13. Völker-Dieben, H.J. *et al.* (2000). Beneficial Effect of HLA-DR Matching On the Survival of Corneal Allografts. *Transplantation*, **70**, 640–648.
14. Reinhard, T. *et al.* (2004). Improvement of Graft Prognosis in Penetrating Normal-Risk Keratoplasty by HLA Class I and II Matching. *Eye*, **18**, 269–277.
15. Vail, A. *et al.* (1994). Influence of Donor and Histocompatibility Factors on Corneal Graft Outcome. *Transplantation*, **58**, 1210–1217.
16. Baggesen, K. *et al.* (1991). HLA-DR/RFLP Compatible Corneal Grafts. *Acta Ophthalmol*, **69**, 229–233.
17. Moore, M.B. *et al.* (1987). Fate of Lyophilized Xenogeneic Corneal Lenticules in Intrastromal Implantation and Epikeratophakia. *Invest Ophthalmol Vis Sci*, **28**, 555–559.
18. Tsai, R.J. and Tseng, S.C (1994). Human Allograft Limbal Transplantation for Corneal Surface Reconstruction. *Cornea*, **13**, 389–400.
19. Pellegrini, G. *et al.* (1997) Long-Term Restoration of Damaged Corneal Surfaces with Autologous Cultivated Corneal Epithelium. *Lancet*, **349**, 990–993.
20. Melles, G.R.J. *et al.* (2002). Sutureless, Posterior Lamellar Keratoplasty: A Case Report of a Modified Technique. *Cornea*, **21**, 325–327.
21. Melles, G.R.J. *et al.* (2006). Descemet Membrane Endothelial Keratoplasty (DMEK). *Cornea*, **25**, 987–990.

10

Small Bowel Transplantation

Christina D. Bali, Vassilios Papalois and Nadey S. Hakim

Many patients die each year lacking a functional small bowel to survive. The minimum amount of small bowel absorptive surface required to sustain life varies from patient to patient. Prolonged survival with oral alimentation alone has been reported in few patients with an intact duodenum and as little as 15 to 45 cm of residual jejunum. However, without long-term total parenteral nutrition (TPN), prolonged patient survival is the exception rather than the rule.[1]

Chronic parenteral nutrition is associated with several complications, including sepsis, venous thrombosis, metabolic disorders and liver dysfunction.[2,3] From studies of patients currently on TPN it would appear that there are between two and three patients per million of population per year who develop irreversible small bowel failure.[4] It is estimated that 20 new patients receiving TPN per year in the UK would be potential candidates for small bowel transplantation.[1] Additionally, the British artificial nutrition survey data shows an increasing annual trend in the adults entering a home TPN treatment programme.[5]

10.1 Indications

The short bowel syndrome comprises the spectrum of conditions resulting from the loss of absolute bowel surface area to loss of appropriate function and is present when the patient is unable to absorb enough nutrients from the intestinal tract to maintain adequate nutrition, health and a feeling of well-being.[4] This may be due to a short bowel following, for example, extensive resection,[6] extensive inflammatory or radiation-induced bowel disease, congenital disease affecting the microvilli of the mucosa, or motility disorders. The short bowel syndrome is the most common pre-transplant diagnosis. The common causes of short bowel syndrome in adults and children are given in Table 10.1.[7]

Three types of intestinal transplantation have been described — isolated intestinal transplantation, combined liver-intestinal grafts and multivisceral graft — in which up to five organs (stomach, duodenum, pancreas, liver, small bowel) are transplanted simultaneously.[8] For the majority of patients, small bowel transplantation is indicated only when surgically irreversible intestinal failure coexists with failure of parenteral nutrition (PN).[8–10] The main causes of PN failure are loss of venous access due to venous thrombosis, PN-related liver disease, and recurrent line related sepsis, especially if the latter is caused by fungus.[8] Proven venous occlusion with availability of either ≤ 2 major neck venous sites with loss of ≥ 1 femoral sites or ≤ 1 major neck venous site and both femoral veins is considered as an indication for

Table 10.1 Causes of intestinal failure.

Adults	Children
Crohn's disease	Intestinal atresia
Superior mesenteric artery thrombosis	Gastroschisis
Superior mesenteric vein thrombosis	Microvillous inclusion disease
Trauma	Necrotizing enterocolitis
Desmoid tumour	Mid-gut volvulus
Volvulus	Chronic intestinal pseudo-obstruction
Radiation enteritis	Crohn's disease
Pseudo-obstruction	

referral of adults to an intestinal transplantation centre. The TPN-induced liver disease is characterized by presence of portal hypertension, cholestasis and cirrhosis.

Paediatric patients with congenital abnormalities of the gastrointestinal tract form the majority of potential candidates for small bowel transplantation.[7] Some of those paediatric patients will have other congenital abnormalities that require careful evaluation to determine whether they are suitable for small bowel transplantation. The intestine is more difficult to transplant than other solid organs due to its strong expression of histocompatibility antigens, large numbers of resident leukocytes, and colonization with microorganisms.[11] Based on the gained experience with solid organ transplantation, small bowel transplantation is contraindicated in the following conditions: marked cardiopulmonary insufficiency, aggressive malignancy, advanced autoimmune diseases, AIDS and existence of life-threatening intra-abdominal or systemic sepsis.[12] There is no upper limit for patients that can undergo intestinal transplantation, although elderly patients are more likely to have other adverse conditions. Likewise, there is no clear lower age limit for paediatric patients. According to the Intestine Transplant Registry data the youngest recipient so far was 1.2 months, and the eldest 67.8 years. Nevertheless, age is included among the factors related to improved patient survival after intestinal transplantation.[13]

10.2 Small Bowel Procurement and Preservation

The small bowel graft should be retrieved from a stable cadaveric heart-beating donor of compatible ABO type. When an isolated intestinal transplant is contemplated (as opposed to a combined liver-intestinal transplant or a multivisceral transplant), care should be taken to ensure a negative lymphocytotoxic crossmatch between donor and recipient.[14]

Factors that may impede transplantation include donor/recipient size incompatibility and cytomegalovirus (CMV) status. Most recipients have had massive bowel resections and thus have heavily scarred abdominal wall from multiple abdominal operations, resulting in reduction of the available space in the peritoneal cavity. Consequently, they often require donors who are 50 to 75% smaller than predicted. This causes a serious problem, especially in infants, which is declared by the high mortality rate on the liver/intestine waiting list (66%) in candidates under six years old.[15] Efforts have been made to surgically resect segments of bowel and/or liver from grafts that would otherwise be too large for the recipient's size.[16]

CMV enteritis is a significant post-transplant complication. Many centres avoid using CMV-positive donors in CMV-negative recipients, thereby excluding many potential donors.[15] Some centres have reported that the administration of an anti-CMV prophylactic treatment to the recipient can act protectively from CMV infections, even if the graft comes from a seropositive CMV donor.[17] The intestinal mucosa is extremely sensitive to ischaemia and hypoxia, secondary to cardiac or respiratory instability of the donor. As a hollow nonsterile organ, the small intestine is very prone to damage, and cold ischaemia times must be minimized. The donor should undergo selective bowel decontamination with antibiotic and antifungal agents given by nasogastric tube. For patients undergoing combined liver and small bowel transplantation, good liver function of the donor is extremely important.

Antilymphocyte preparations, to prevent graft-versus-host disease, have been used in some centres.[18,19] More recently, lymphocyte depletion of the graft by *ex vivo* intestine irradiation has been applied, but there are still concerns about the graft radiation damage.[20]

For the retrieval operation the donor is heparinized and the supraceliac aorta cross-clamped. In adults, a litre of cold University of Wisconsin (UW) solution is infused into the aorta, and another litre of UW into the portal vein, venting the vena cava either into the chest or through a cannula into an iliac vein. Excessive perfusion may damage the intestinal graft. Appropriately smaller volumes of perfusate should be administered to paediatric donors. The abdominal cavity is packed with ice slush to assist the cooling. If both of the small bowel and liver are to be used for separate isolated transplants, the liver and the intestine can be retrieved en bloc and separated at the back table.[21] The cadaveric graft is based on the superior mesenteric artery (SMA) with an aortic (Carrel) patch and the superior mesenteric/proximal portal vein (PV). In the case that the graft is retrieved from a live donor it is based on distal SMA and SMV, and it is consisted of one third of the donor's small bowel.[8]

10.3 Recipient Operation

The allograft artery is anastomosed directly around the orifice of the recipient's SMA or to the abdominal aorta with the Carrel patch. The SMV/PV are anastomosed to either the right side of the recipient's portal vein, which can be approached just behind the bile duct after the mobilization of duodenum and head of the pancreas, or more simply to the anterior surface of the inferior vena cava (IVC) at the same level as the arterial anastomosis to the aorta.

Intestinal continuity is restored by performing a proximal side-to-side anastomosis to the remaining recipient gut. The graft ileus is anastomosed to the recipient's remaining small or large bowel. A distal ileostomy (chimney or Mickulitz type) is also fashioned to permit frequent endoscopic and histologic monitoring of the intestine graft. This ileostomy can be closed if the graft function has been secured. The venous drainage of clusters of organs that include the liver flows into the recipient vena cava via a direct anastomosis or patch of donor vena cava. Any residual recipient viscera are anastomosed into the vena cava to form a porta-caval shunt or "piggy–backed" onto the portal vein of the liver/intestinal graft. Biliary drainage of the liver is restored either by a direct anastomosis to the stump of the native bile duct or to a Roux loop created from the transplanted bowel. A feeding gastrostomy or jejunostomy catheter is placed to provide continuous enteral feeding.

The previously scarred abdominal wall and the post-reperfusion graft oedema are two factors that adversely affect the abdominal closure after small intestine transplantation. Except from the aforementioned graft reduction techniques, relaxing fasciotomy, use of muscle or skin flaps and even abdominal wall transplantation have been utilized to deal with this really difficult problem.[16,22]

10.4 Post-Operative Management

10.4.1 Intensive care unit

Well-nourished patients may be extubated 24 to 48 hours after surgery, whereas malnourished patients often require a longer period of ventilation.

A Duplex ultrasonography scan is usually necessary for the assessment of vascular patency of the graft. Prophylactic antibiotic treatment is started to cover for any potential bacterial, fungal or viral infection. Treatment with prostaglandin E1, which is used for its beneficial effects on the microcirculation, is initiated.[23]

Fluid losses from stoma, faeces, jejunal and gastric tubes, and abdominal drains must be closely monitored and replaced. The small bowel graft may become oedematous during the early post–operative period with fluid sequestration into the tissues, which later are released back into the circulation. Early graft viability can be assessed by observing the colour of the intestine mucosa of the ileostomy, and, if necessary, an endoscopic evaluation can also be performed.

10.4.2 Immunosuppression

The immunosuppressive therapy for the intestinal transplantation is based on tacrolimus (FK), a calcineurin inhibitor. FK is administered to achieve a trough level of 15 to 20 ng/mL by the end of the first post–operative week (dose of 0.2 to 0.3 mg/kg per day), and levels are generally tapered to between 5 and 10 mg/L by the end of the first year.[14] Steroids are also administered typically at 20 mg per day for adults and 0.3 mg/kg per day for children.

The current policy is to avoid combination maintenance therapy with adjunctive agents. Monotherapy with tacrolimus following induction with lymphocyte depleting antibodies (ATG, Campath 1H, OKT3) or with monoclonal anti–IL-2 receptor antibodies (dacluzimab) is the most preferred therapeutic model. The advantages of antibody pre-conditioning include less potent maintenance immunosuppression and improved tolerance; though it permits the administration of lower tacrolimus dose.[8]

10.4.3 Monitoring of rejection

Clinical observation, endoscopic examination and bowel biopsies are used to monitor small bowel graft rejection. Clinical features that correlate well with histologic rejection are sudden onset of fever, abdominal distention ileus, increased ileostomy output, haematemesis, stomal bleeding and discoloration of stoma. Septicaemia due to gut-derived organisms correlates strongly with intestinal rejection. Endoscopy is performed once or twice weekly for the first post-operative month.[24] Over the next five months the frequency of endoscopy is reduced to once every three or four weeks, or more frequently if indicated. Prompt histological diagnosis and treatment is usually effective to prevent severe rejection. In most cases acute rejection occurs within the first post-operative trimester, but can occur more than a year after transplantation. Acute rejection is usually steroid responsive whereas antilymphocyte antibodies can also be effectively used.[8] If severe rejection is diagnosed the only life-saving treatment is to perform graft enterectomy.[25]

The earliest endoscopic signs of rejection are oedema, erythaema and aperistalsis. More advanced rejection is characterized by aphthous ulcers. Severe rejection is marked by broad-based ulcers or completely denuded mucosa, sometimes covered by pseudomembranes. Acute cellular rejection is marked by the presence of activated lymphocytes attacking the crypt epithelium to produce cryptitis.[26] Apoptosis of crypt cells then occurs. Untreated rejection leads to complete endothelial sloughing, which results in pseudomembranous enteritis. Chronic rejection has become more important as effective medical treatments for acute rejection have been discovered. The incidence of chronic rejection is approximately 8%. Chronic rejection is usually difficult to detect, resulting in delayed diagnosis and treatment. The clinical presentation consists of watery diarrhoea, abdominal pain and weight loss. In order to make a histological diagnosis the intestinal wall biopsies should be of full thickness. In chronic rejection the histological changes lay deep in the bowel wall and affect the vasculature. The mucosa layer may show no specific changes. The pathological feature of chronic rejection is obliterative endarteropathy with neointimal hyperplasia.[27]

Currently, two new methods are being studied regarding early diagnosis of rejection: the zoom video endoscopy (ZVE) and the measurement of plasma levels of citrulline. ZVE is the use of a magnifying endoscope that has the ability to distinguish early mucosal changes of rejection better than a conventional endoscope.[28] Citrulline, an amino acid, has been found to be an accurate biomarker of rejection, since its plasma levels are proportional to the intestinal function.[29]

10.4.4 Infections

In the post-transplantation period, infection is the leading cause of morbidity and mortality in the intestine transplant recipient, accounting for up to 70% of deaths. Bacterial, viral or fungal infections can be the pathogenic microorganisms. Fatal septic infections are often polymicrobial and associated with multisystem organ failure. Factors predisposing to the occurrence of infection are the required higher levels of immunosuppression, the prolonged operative time with a technically difficult surgery, the severity of pre-operative liver disease, sepsis prior to transplantation, malnutrition, transfusions, the inability to close the abdominal wall, technical complications (anastomotic leaks) and multiple invasive lines, catheters and drains.[30]

Infection is more common during rejection episodes because of the need to increase immunosuppression, as well as the bacterial translocation associated with loss of mucosal integrity. Viral infections such as cytomegalovirus and Epstein–Barr virus are especially problematic. CMV is the most common viral pathogen following intestine transplantation, with an overall incidence of 34%.[30] Infection with EBV remains one of the most serious problems of immunosuppressive management in transplantation. EBV-associated post-transplant lymphoproliferative disorders (PTLD) comprise a range of disorders from non-specific viral illness to lymphoma. The incidence of PTLD is higher with intestinal transplant recipients, especially in the paediatric population, and consist a major cause of death — the mortality rate is 45 to 50%.[30]

10.4.5 Graft–versus–host disease (GvHD)

The large quantity of lymphoid tissue present in the mesenteric lymph nodes, Peyer's patches and lamina propria of the intestinal graft can be activated against the recipient. Although it was initially believed that intestine transplantation would carry a high risk for GvHD, the incidence is 6 to 16% in the most active intestine transplant centres.[8] The most common clinical presentation of GvHD is an erythematous, maculopapular rash that usually affects the palms, soles, ears and trunk. Symptoms of fever, diarrhoea, malaisia and pancytopenia may also be present. Histologic criteria include keratinocyte necrosis, epithelial apoptosis of the native GI tract or epithelial necrosis of the oral mucosa.[31] Although GvHD has been fatal in a very few cases, the majority have been self-limiting with spontaneous resolution.

10.5 Intestinal Function

Small bowel motility usually recovers within 24 to 48 hours post transplant. Intestinal function after transplantation is reduced by denervation, lymphatic disruption, ischemic injury, acute rejection and the effects of immunosuppressive drugs.[32]

Absorption is a good indicator of satisfactory function of the transplanted intestine and is gauged by measuring the volume and composition of the stoma effluent. The most useful indicators are the carbohydrate and fat absorption. The first is assessed with the D-xylose test and the presence of reducing substances. If the D-xylose test is abnormal, the contingence of rejection should be ruled out. After the first month the carbohydrate absorption is present.[30] Once carbohydrate absorption has been established, peptide solutions can be introduced and nitrogen balance determined. Fat absorption is presented later because of the disruption of lymphatic vessels of the intestine. Evaluation of fat absorption can be performed by estimating the difference between fat intake and output through the 24-hour faecal fat load. During the first post-transplant period most of the lipid calories are administrated intravenously. Fat in the form of medium-chain triglycerides is added gradually to the enteral diet as the fat malabsorption diminishes over time.

The incidence of diarrhoea is high following small intestinal transplantation. This may be attributed to rapid transit associated with denervation of the intestinal graft, to bacterial overgrowth, to malabsorption or to the loss of the ileocecal valve. In the absence of rejection, patients with high stomal output should be treated with antidiarrhoeal medications in order to reduce enteral losses and possibility of dehydration. Another option is to include in the intestinal graft the ileocecal valve and part of the right colon, which is anastomosed to the recipient's large bowel.[24]

10.6 Results of Small Bowel Transplantation

According to the report of the Intestinal Transplant Registry, the small bowel transplantation has become the definitive treatment of patients with chronic intestinal failure, who cannot be maintained on parenteral nutrition. During the last decade the cases of intestinal transplantation per year have been doubled. Isolate intestine transplants performed were more common in adults (55%) as compared with paediatric recipients (37%). Conversely, paediatric recipients received combined intestinal and liver transplants more often than adults (50% and 21%, respectively). Approximately 3% of the grafts were obtained from live donors.[13]

With the advance of immunosuppressive therapy the outcome of intestinal transplantation has been improved over the last decade. The one-year patient/graft survival rates is reported to be 77%/65% for intestinal grafts, 60%/59% for combined intestinal-liver grafts, and 66%/61% for multivisceral grafts.[13] The difference between patient and graft survival is related to the ability of removing the graft in case of rejection (the commonest indication), thrombosis/ischaemia or bleeding, and uncontrollable sepsis.[33] One-year graft/patient survivals were significantly better in patients who were waiting at home instead of being in the hospital. The most common causes of death in transplant recipients were sepsis (46.0%), rejection (11.2%), respiratory causes (6.6%), technical problems (6.2%) and lymphoma (6.2%).[13,33] Lymphoproliferative disease is a major cause of post-operative mortality and it is most frequent in the paediatric population. Grant et al. report that, of the patients who were alive for more than six months post transplant, 81% were off total parenteral nutrition (TPN), 3.9% required IV fluids only, 6.4% required partial TPN and 7.9% were TPN-dependent after their graft was removed.[13] Comparative studies between long-term TPN and intestinal transplantation regarding the quality of life showed equal or better quality in transplanted patients.[33]

Small bowel transplantation can be a life-saving procedure for patients with irreversible intestinal failure who develop complications from TPN. Early referral of those patients for intestinal transplantation is vital for better outcome. The field of small bowel transplantation is moving and improving rapidly over time. Further research in the immunosuppression area and post-operative management of complications is needed before intestinal transplantation can become the treatment of choice for intestinal failure.

References

1. Sarr, M.G. and Hakim, N.S. (1994). In Sarr, M.G. and Hakim, N.S. (eds), *Enteric Physiology of the Transplanted Intestine*, Landes, Austin, Texas, pp. 3–7.

2. Quigley, E.M. *et al.* (1993). Hepatobiliary Complications of Total Parenteral Nutrition, *Gastroenterology*, **104**, 286–301.

3. Messing, B. *et al.* (1999). Long-Term Survival and Parenteral Nutrition Dependence in Adult Patients with Short Bowel Syndrome, *Gastroenterology*, **117**, 1043–1050.

4. Lennard-Jones, J.E. (1990). Indications and Need for Long-Term Parenteral Nutrition: Implications for Intestinal Transplantation, *Transplant Proc*, **24**, 2427–2429.

5. Glencorse, C. *et al.* (British Artificial Nutrition Survey report) (2005). *Trends in Artificial Nutritional Support in the UK Between 1996 and 2002*. Available at http://www.bapen.org.uk/pdfs/exec_summ9602.pdf (accessed 22 June 2011).

6. Hancock, B.J. and Wiseman, N.E. (1990). Lethal Short-Bowel Syndrome, *J Pediatr Surg*, **25**, 1131–1134.

7. Mittal, N.K. *et al.* (2000). Current Indications for Intestinal Transplantation, *Curr Opin Org Transplant*, **5**, 279–283.

8. Middleton, S.J. and Jamieson, N.V. (2005). The Current Status of Small Bowel Transplantation in the UK and Internationally, *Gut*, **54**, 1650–1657.

9. Ingham Clark, C.I. *et al.* (1992). Potential Candidates for Small Bowel Transplantation, *Brit J Surg*, **79**, 676–679.

10. Thompson, J.S. (1990). Recent Advances in the Surgical Treatment of the Short-Bowel Syndrome, *Surg Annu*, **22**, 107–127.

11. Newell, K.A. (2003). Transplantation of the Intestine: Is it Truly Different? *Am J Transplant*, **3**, 1–2.

12. Abu-Elmagd, K. and Bond, G. (2003). Gut Failure and Abdominal Visceral Transplantation, *Proc Nutr Soc*, **62**, 727–737.

13. Grant, D. *et al.* (2003). Report of the Intestine Transplant Registry, *Ann Surg*, **241**, 607–613.

14. Al-Hussaini, A., Tredger, M.J. and Dhawan, A. (2005). Immunosuppression in Pediatric Liver and Intestinal Transplantation: A Closer Look at the Arsenal, *J Pediatr Gastr Nutr*, **41**, 152–165.

15. Goulet, O. *et al.* (2004). Irreversible Intestinal Failure, *J Pediatr Gastr Nutr*, **38**, 250–269.

16. de Ville de Goyer, J. *et al.* (2000). En Bloc Combined Reduced Liver and Small Bowel Transplants: From Large Donors to Small Children, *Transplantation*, **69**, 555–559.

17. Tzakis, A.G. (2001). Cytomegalovirus Prophylaxis with Gancyclovir and Cytomegalovirus Immune Globulin in Liver and Intestinal Transplantation, *Transpl Infect Dis*, **3**, 35–39.

18. Diflo, T. *et al.* (1988). The Effects of Antilymphocyte Serum and Cyclosporine on Orthotopic Small Bowel Allografts in the Rat, *Transplant Proc*, **20**, 200–202.

19. Grant, D. *et al.* (1990). Graft-versus-Host Disease after Clinical Small Bowel/Liver Transplantation, *Transplant Proc*, **22**, 2464.

20. Murase, N. *et al.* (1999). Immunomodulation of Intestinal Transplant with Allograft Irradiation and Simultaneous Donor Bone Marrow Infusion, *Transplant Proc,* **31**, 565–566.
21. Casavilla, A. *et al.* (1992). Logistics and Technique for Combined Hepatic-Intestinal Retrieval, *Ann Surg,* **216**, 605–609.
22. Levi, D.M. *et al.* (2003). Transplantation of the Abdominal Wall, *Lancet,* **361**, 2173–2176.
23. Langnas, A.N. (2004). Advances in Small Intestine Transplantation, *Transplantation,* **77**, S75–S78.
24. Tzakis, A.G. *et al.* (1993). Piggyback Orthotopic Intestinal Transplantation, *Surg Gynecol Obstet,* **176**, 297–298.
25. Kato, T. *et al.* (2000). Is Severe Rejection an Indication for Retransplantation? *Transplant Proc,* **32**, 1201.
26. Abu-Elmagd, K.M. *et al.* (1993). Monitoring and Treatment of Intestinal Allograft Rejection in Humans, *Transplant Proc,* **25**, 1202–1203.
27. Lee, R.G. *et al.* (1996). Pathology of Human Intestinal Transplantation, *Gastroenterology,* **110**, 1820–1834.
28. Kato, T. *et al.* (2000). Improved Rejection Surveillance in Intestinal Transplant Recipients With Frequent Use of Zoom Video Endoscopy, *Transplant Proc,* **32**, 1200.
29. Pappas, P.A. *et al.* (2004). An Analysis of the Association Between Serum Citrulline and Acute Rejection Among 26 Recipients of Intestinal Transplant, *Am J Transplant,* **4**, 1124–1132.
30. Kosmach Park, B. (2002). Intestine Transplantation, *Organ Transplant,* available at: http://www.medscape.com/viewarticle/436543 (accessed 22 February 2005).
31. Reyes, J. and Abu-Elmagd, K. (1999). 'Small Bowel and Liver Transplantation in Children', in Kelly, D.A. (ed), *Diseases of the Biliary System in Children,* Blackwell Science, Osney Mead, Oxford, pp. 313–331.
32. Dionigi, P., Alessiani, M. and Ferrazi, A. (2001). Irreversible Intestinal Failure, Nutrition Support, and Small Bowel Transplantation, *Nutrition* **17**, 747–750.
33. Fryer, J.P. (2005). Intestinal Transplantation: An Update, *Curr Opin Gastroenterol,* **21**, 162–168.

11

Haemopoietic Stem Cell Transplantation

Shaun R. McCann

11.1 Historical Perspective

Interest in bone marrow transplantation (BMT) was stimulated because of atomic weapons and the devastating effects of ionising radiation. A number of important observations, including Jacobson's demonstration of the protective effect of splenic shielding on lethally irradiated mice, laid the groundwork for human bone marrow transplantation.[1] By the late 1950s it became clear that the protective effect of spleen or marrow depended on the presence of a cellular component, which was subsequently shown to be the so-called pluripotent stem cell. The existence of the pluripotent stem cell in the animal model and the development of clonogenic assays for haemopoietic progenitors and stem cells was of great significance in the understanding of the mechanisms underlying bone marrow transplantation.

In 1970, Bortin reviewed 203 cases of human transplantation and showed that there were only 11 in whom there was unequivocal evidence of sustained donor engraftment, and only three of them were alive at the time of the report.[2] When one considers the lack of understanding of the histocompatibility complex (HLA, MHC) it is not surprising that the initial results were so poor. The publication by Thomas *et al.* in 1975 showing the efficacy of allogeneic BMT in the treatment of acute leukaemia provided the stimulus for a rapid development of BMT units throughout the world.[3] By 2005 the Centre for International Blood Transplant and Marrow Research (CIBMTR) had registered 388 teams in 44 countries. Between 1968 and 2005 the registry had received data on 97,454 allogeneic and 89,752 autologous transplants.

11.2 Biological Perspective

The quest to identify and purify the true pluripotent human haemopoietic stem cell is not yet complete; however, a number of claims can be made. It is clear that the pluripotent stem cell resides in the mononuclear cell fraction of the bone marrow.[4] Small numbers of pluripotent stem cell circulate and the number of stem cells in the circulation can be significantly influenced by the administration of chemotherapeutic agents and/or growth factors.[5] A combination of clonogenic assays and surface 'antigen' profiles is used to identify and quantify progenitors. Short-term cultures support the growth of unipotent progenitors and more immature multipotent progenitors can be assayed using the CFU-GEMM (CFU-mix) assay.[6] The assay which approximates most closely to the pluripotent stem cell in the human being is the long-term culture initiating cell assay (LT-CIC).[7] CD34 is a cell-surface glycophosphoprotein expressed on early lymphohaemopoietic stem cells and progenitors. The CD-34 surface antigen is found on haemopoietic stem cells in bone marrow (BM), mobilised peripheral blood mononuclear cells (PBSC) and umbilical cord mononuclear cells (UCB). The measurement of the CD34 positive population of cells is carried out by flow cytometry and there are a number of internationally recognised quality assurance schemes for the measurement of CD34. The recommended cut-off for the number of CD34+ cells in allogeneic PBSC transplantation is $4.0 - 6.0 \times 10^6/kg$, in autologous PBSC is $2.5 - 4.0 \times 10^6/kg$ (varies) for different diseases and in UCB is $1.7 \times 1^5/kg$. CD34+ plays a role in stem cell/progenitor localisation/adhesion in the bone marrow.[8]

11.3 Practicalities of Bone Marrow Transplantation

11.3.1 Allogeneic stem cell transplantation (Allo SCT)

The basic approach to Allo SCT is shown in Figure 11.1. In patients with acute leukaemia (AL) there are a number of major issues. The conditioning

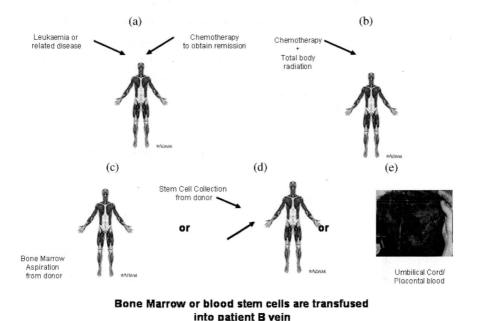

(a) (b)

Leukaemia or related disease → Chemotherapy to obtain remission

Chemotherapy + Total body radiation

(c) (d) (e)

Stem Cell Collection from donor

or

or

Bone Marrow Aspiration from donor

Umbilical Cord/ Placental blood

Bone Marrow or blood stem cells are transfused into patient B vein

Figure 11.1 Allogeneic stem cell transplantation. The patient is treated until remission is obtained, and then receives myeloablative conditioning therapy (chemo/radiotherapy or chemotherapy alone). Bone marrow is collected from the donor's pelvis under general anaesthesia and infused into the recipient via a right atrial catheter.

therapy (Cyclophosphamide and total body irradiation TBI or Busulphan PO or IV and Cyclophosphamide are the two most commonly used preparative regimens) is required to have an anti-leukaemic effect and also to eradicate all host haematopoiesis in order to 'make space' for the donor marrow; however, residual host haematopoietic cells may coexist with donor cells following Allo SCT. This is known as mixed chimaerism and its influence on leukaemia relapse or graft rejection has been reviewed.[9]

The anti-leukaemic effect of the conditioning therapy is augmented by the allogeneic or graft-versus-leukaemia (GvL) effect. It has been traditional to carry out bone marrow transplantation for AL at a time when the recipient is in 'complete remission', i.e. when the presumed burden of residual leukaemia is minimal. Many newer regimens are currently under investigation to see if the 'tumour cell kill' can be increased; however, toxicity of chemotherapeutic regimens continues to be a dose-limiting factor.

Increasing irradiation doses will result in a decreased leukaemia relapse rate but unfortunately overall survival is not increased because of increased transplant related mortality (TRM).[10] In severe aplastic anaemia (SAA) and other non-malignant disorders the primary role of the conditioning irradiation is not recommended for patients with non-malignant haematopoietic diseases undergoing Allo SCT because of long-term toxicity.

11.3.2 Non-myeloablative stem cell (reduced intensity conditioning) transplantation

Because of the overwhelming toxicity of myeloablative conditioning therapy and its contribution to TRM and morbidity, other approaches have more recently been tested. The philosophical view has been altered to try to increase the graft-versus-leukaemia (GvL) effect and to rely more intensely on immunosuppression of the recipient to prevent graft rejection. So-called 'non-myeloablative' or reduced-intensity transplantation is gaining in popularity (Figure 11.2).

The preparative regimens are varied but consist of potent immunosuppression with purine analogues or ATG combined with chemotherapy or total body irradiation. These regimens are associated with a marked reduction in transplant-related toxicity, morbidity and mortality, and have widened the scope of transplant to include older patients and patients with co-morbidity (which might have previously precluded them from consideration for allogeneic transplantation). As yet there has been no large-scale prospective randomised clinical trial in subgroups of patients directly comparing myeloablative with non-myeloablative regimens. However, encouraging results in terms of disease-free survival have been reported for diseases such as acute myeloid leukaemia.[11] Non-myeloablative or reduced intensity preparatory regimens are usually accompanied by a transplantation of mobilised peripheral blood stem cells (PBSC), as opposed to bone marrow cells.

11.4 Haemopoietic Chimaerism

In the majority of recipients there is a combination of host and donor haemopoeisis for some time after transplantation (mixed haemopoietic chimaerism). Over time the majority of patients will convert to complete

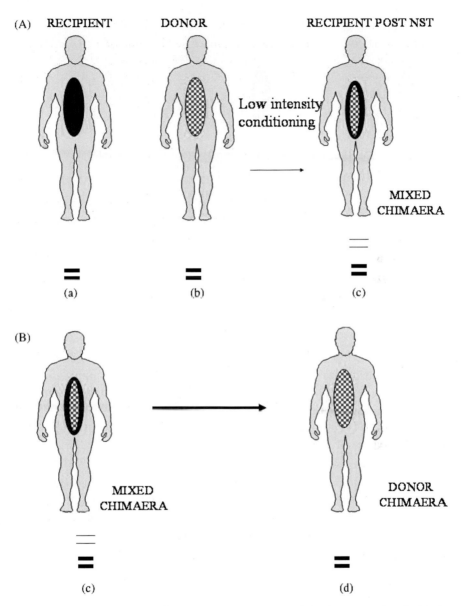

Figure 11.2 (A) Non–myeloablative stem cell transplantation. Peripheral blood–mobilised stem cells are infused into the patient after non-myeloablative conditioning and potent immunosuppressive therapy. (B) Evolution to donor chimaerism. Over time, all the stem cells in the recipient are donor in type (a donor chimaera). This can be measured using differences in DNA profile between host and donor.

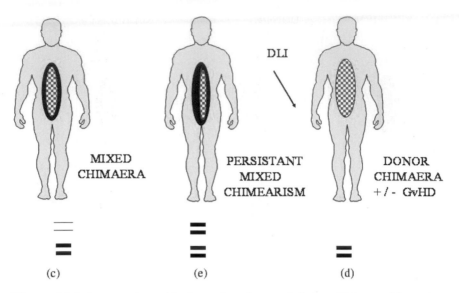

Figure 11.3 Intervention with donor lymphocyte infusion. If donor chimaerism does not occur an infusion of 'donor lymphocytes' is given to the patient.

donor chimaeras but in the event of a failure to achieve complete donor chimaerism the use of donor lymphocyte infusions (DLI) may be considered (Figure 11.3).[12]

11.5 Choice of Donor

The ideal donor is a family member, sharing the same class I (A,B,C) and II (DR) histocompatibility (HLA) antigen profile. Because HLA antigens are inherited as a haplotype from each parent there is an approximately 1:4 chance of each sibling sharing the same HLA type. The chances of finding a compatible sibling donor therefore largely reflect family size. Thus, in most countries (with some exceptions), there is a 1:3 chance of finding a compatible sibling.[13,14] In the absence of a compatible sibling an extended family search probably increases the chance of finding a donor by a further 5%. The availability of an identical twin donor may seem ideal; however, numerous studies have demonstrated a significantly higher rate of leukaemia relapse. Because of these difficulties a search for a 'matched' donor from a pool of unrelated individual volunteers (MVUD) has become increasingly frequent.

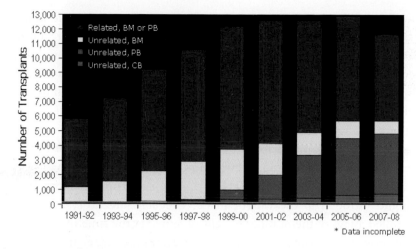

Figure 11.4 Allogeneic transplants in patients under 20 years, by donor type and graft source, registered with CIBMR, 1991 to 2008. Increasing numbers of unrelated stem cell transplants over time. (Reproduced with kind permission of the CIBMTR.)

A large number of registries exist and a search of such registries may increase the chance of finding a donor by up to 90%. Initially, MVUD donors were used only if they were a full phenotypic match, but data from Beatty *et al.* indicates that there are certain situations where a so-called 'permissible mismatch' may be used successfully.[15] The widespread use of molecular methods of typing has ensured more precise matching between donor/recipient pairs and therefore better outcome. Clinical results have exceeded expectations in patients receiving MVUD Allo SCT for leukaemia and the number of unrelated donor transplants continues to increase (Figure 11.4).[16] However, the contribution of MVUD to SAA remains problematical with major problems of graft rejection. The use of non-myeloablative (or reduced-intensity conditioning) transplants together with good molecular typing may in the future improve the outcome for these patients.

11.6 Autologous Stem Cell Transplantation

Another approach to the absence of compatible sibling is to use mobilised peripheral blood stem cells (PBSC) or bone marrow stem cells from the patient. Mobilised PBSC are used in the majority of autograft situations as outlined. Problems include difficulty in harvesting adequate numbers of stem cells because of prior chemo-radiotherapy and the possibility of harvesting tumour cells which when re-infused will contribute to disease relapse. The contribution of such cells to relapse has been documented in acute and chronic leukaemias.[17] *In vitro* treatment of the stem cells, so-called 'purging', is no longer commonly used. Likewise, the use of *in vitro* drug therapy to eradicate residual tumour cells hare largely fallen out of favour. Important issues at the time of collection of PBSC or bone marrow cells for autografting include sterility at the time of collection, adequate storage in liquid nitrogen in the vapour phase, excellent inventory and quality-controlled assays of the number of cells obtained at the time of harvest, and re-infusion. Regulations governing the collection, storage and re-infusion of PBSC and bone marrow cells have been published by JACIE[18] and are the subject of an EU directive.[19]

11.7 Blood Versus Marrow Versus Umbilical Cord Blood (UCB)

Adequate numbers of progenitors to sustain long-term haemopoesis can be mobilised into the circulation following chemotherapy (e.g. cyclophosphamide) and/or growth factors such as recombinant granulocyte colony stimulating factor (rh-G-CSF) or recombinant granulocyte macrophage stimulating factor (rh-GMCSF).[5] This can be achieved in patients in spite of evidence of severe marrow damage. Growth factors have also been used to mobilise progenitor cells from volunteer donors for allogeneic (PBSC) transplants.[20] Mononuclear cells can subsequently be collected using a cell separator (Figure 11.5).

Mobilising PBSCs avoids the use of a general anaesthetic, which is required for marrow harvest. Issues concerning the use of PBSC mobilised from volunteer donors include the administration of growth factors to normal individuals (rare cases of splenic rupture and fear of possible leukaemogenicity), the difference in the composition of the mononuclear cell component compared to marrow (the fear of an increased incidence of graft–versus–host disease [GvHD]; see 11.9.4), preservation of the GvL effect and the ability of the PBSC to establish long-term haematopoiesis in the

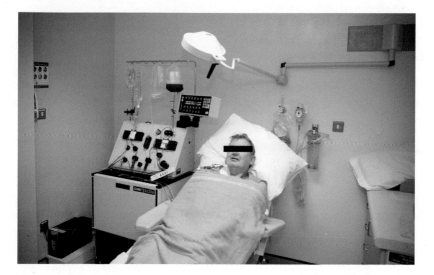

Figure 11.5 Collecting mobilised peripheral blood stem cells from a patient/donor using a cell separator.

allogeneic setting. The latter fear has been allayed and confidence in the ability of PBSC to achieve long-term stable engraftment can be judged by the change in the name of the European Group for Bone Marrow Transplantation (EBMT) to the European Group for Blood and Marrow Transplantation in 1994.

Umbilical cord blood (CB) is an important source of haemopoietic stem cells. The number of cells collected at the time of delivery is usually less than 100 ml, thereby limiting its usefulness for SCT primarily to children. The first CB transplant (UCBT) was performed in 1998 in a patient with Fanconi anaemia.[21] The patient is alive and well at the time of writing. The requirement for HLA matching in UCBT is much less stringent compared to marrow or PBSC and there is no requirement for high resolution typing for HLA,-B,-C, -DRB1 or DQB1.[22] To date, over 6,000 patients have received UCBT. The number of nucleated cells infused per kg should be 2×10^7, and CD34+ cells 2×10^5. The incidence of cGVHD after unrelated HLA-mismatched UCBT in children and adults is reduced compared to unrelated unmanipulated HLA-identical BMT and similar to an unrelated HLA-matched T–cell-depleted BMT.

11.8 Clinical Results

11.8.1 Leukaemia

The results of long-term survival of recipients of Allo SCT for acute leukaemia have been widely published by the CIBMTR and the EMMT and other large registries. Long-term leukaemia-free survival following Allo SCT depends to a large extent on the stage of the disease at the time of transplantation. Outcomes of an Allo SCT for acute leukaemia show long-term survival figures of between 40 and 60%. Causes of death can be divided between 'transplant-related mortality' (TRM), GvHD and leukaemia relapse. TRM refers to complications such as pulmonary and cardiac toxicity of cyclophosphamide, haemorrhagic cystitis and sinusoidal-obstructive syndrome of the liver (SOS, VOD). Infection and mucosal bowel injury still remain major clinical problems. Acute GvHD may be a cause of early mortality (within the first three months) in spite of aggressive prophylaxis with drugs such as cyclosporin and/or methotrexate and tacrolimus (FK-506). Chronic GvHD occurs classically more than a hundred days after Allo SCT and is usually associated with death from infection. The use of mobilised PBSC instead of bone marrow cells for Allo SCT is associated with an increased of chronic GvHD although the risk of leukaemia relapse appears to be decreased, although this is controversial.[23,24] Leukaemia relapse may occur any time after Allo SCT. The majority of relapses occur within the first year although late relapses have been reported. A small number of deaths are attributable to secondary tumours,[25] most CNS, which are presumed to be caused by the conditioning therapy. In rare cases leukaemia relapse has been documented in cells of donor origin.[26]

11.8.2 Chronic myeloid leukaemia (CML)

Until the year 2000, chronic myeloid leukaemia (CML) was the major indication for Allo SCT in Europe and North America. The advent of imatinib mesylate (Glivec), a tyrosine kinase (TK) inhibitor and the demonstration by Brian Druker[27] and colleagues that administration of this agent could result in complete karyotypic remission in patients with CML has dramatically altered the role of Allo SCT in this disease (Figure 11.6). CML has now become one of the least frequent indications for Allo SCT and the

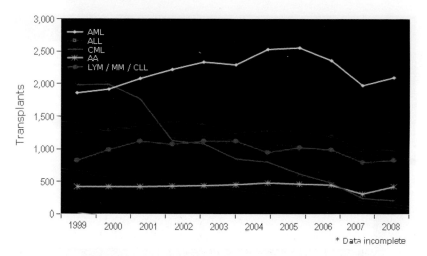

Figure 11.6 Number of allogeneic transplants by disease, registered with CIBMTR, 1998 to 2000. The number of patients with CML receiving stem cell transplants has decreased over time since the introduction of tyrosine kinase inhibition. (Reproduced with kind permission of the CIBMTR.)

role of other TK inhibitors, used alone or in combination with imatinib, is under current investigation. At the moment, sibling Allo SCT or MVUD is confined to patients who have become resistant to imatinib or who have accelerated or blast crisis disease in whom no other modality of therapy has been shown to be curative. The long-term implications of the use of TK inhibitors in CML is as yet unknown and the role of Allo SCT may again become more important in patients who develop resistance and/or progressive disease five, ten or fifteen years following their initial response. Initial evidence does not suggest a deleterious effect of imatinib administered to patients prior to Allo SCT.[28]

11.8.3 Severe aplastic anaemia (SAA)

For young patients with SAA the advent of BMT has completely changed their outcome. A disease that previously had an 80% mortality rate in the first three months now has a long-term survival of 60 to 80% (Figure 11.7). Unlike leukaemia, mortality is clearly linked to age with patients over 30 years having a significantly poorer outlook following BMT.[29] The last ten years have seen dramatic improvements in SAA outcome following

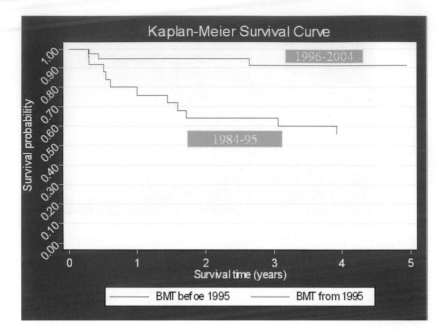

Figure 11.7 Kaplan–Meier survival curve. Improved survival of patients in St James's Hospital, Dublin, following allogeneic bone marrow transplantation for severe aplastic anaemia over time.

immunosuppressive therapy (IT) with antithymocyte globulin (ATG). This modality has been so successful that some investigators recommend a trial of IT prior to Allo SCT in recipients over 30 years. Unlike leukaemia, the ideal donor for a patient with SAA is an identical twin as there is no question of relapse of a malignant process.

11.8.4 Thalassaemia and other non-malignant conditions

Results in a large series of patients from Italy indicate that patients who have been regularly chelated and do not have liver disease have a 94% chance of being cured of β Thalassaemia.[30] Numbers of patients with homozygous sickle–cell disease who have undergone SCT remain small and this therapeutic option should only be considered for selected young patients with severe morbidity due to their disease. Successful outcome of SCT for Gaucher's disease and a number of metabolic disorders has been reported. This clinical outcome depends on the patient's age at the time of SCT and the presence of CNS involvement. The first successful BMT for severe combined immune deficiency was reported in 1969. In Europe the cure rate has been in excess of 93% since 1983.[31]

11.8.5 Autologous grafting

Autografting has gained widespread popularity in the last ten years, particularly for diseases such as Hodgkin's lymphoma (HL), non-Hodgkin's lymphoma (NHL) and multiple myeloma (MM). As indicated previously, many individuals requiring Allo SCT will not have a compatible donor. Relapsing/responsive NHL and HD are particularly amenable to autografting and this is now considered the treatment of choice by investigators.[32] The role of autografting in MM has been extremely successful in achieving prolonged remission, although not cure, in many patients. A seminal randomised trial leading to the more widespread acceptance of autografting in MM was published by the IFM French myeloma group in 1996.[33] High-dose therapy was associated with a five-year overall survival rate of 52% compared to 10% in the conventional chemotherapy group. The superiority of Allo SCT in terms of progression-free survival and overall survival has since been confirmed by many other centres and high-dose treatment with autologous stem cell transplantation has now become the standard of care for patients with MM below the age of 65 years. The use of a second autograft in tandem or with reduced-intensity allograft for patients with MM is currently under investigation.

11.9 Clinical Problems

11.9.1 Engraftment

Animal data indicate that a dose of $1 - 2 \times 10^8$/kg mononuclear cells is required for stable engraftment,[34] and this is the aim of transplant teams. Graft failure/rejection following SCT for leukaemia occurs in under 5% of cases.[35] Graft failure/rejection is a problem, however, in recipients of an SCT for SAA.[36] Graft rejection rates in SAA have been reduced from 32% in the mid 1970s to 8% in the 1990s. This reduction has been coincidental with the introduction of cyclosporine.[37] Long-term survival has been shown by

EBMT to have increased significantly since 1995 in patients receiving SCT for SAA. Current studies are underway to investigate the role of unrelated donors and reduced-intensity conditioning for the treatment of patients in whom a sibling donor is not a possibility for patients with SAA. Mobilised PBSC are the stem cells of choice for patients undergoing auto grafting and in many patients undergoing allogeneic SCT. Randomised trials have shown conclusively that PBSC in the allogeneic setting are associated with an increased risk of chronic graft-versus-host disease (cGvHD). However, relapse rates for leukaemia have also decreased. Currently, many centres advocate the use of PBSC in the allogeneic setting for patients with high-risk leukaemia in an effort to maximise the graft-versus-leukaemia effect (GvL). PBSC continues to be the preferred source of stem cells in patients undergoing reduced-intensity allografting.

11.9.2 Support care and growth factors

Support care, including growth factors and haematology support, has been an intrinsic part of the success story of SCT. These factors include the liberal use of allogeneic platelet and red cell concentrates, and plasma derivatives (all cellular blood products are irradiated prior to infusion to prevent GvHD). Filtration of cellular blood products to remove leukocytes is also recommended and may have the dual effect of reducing non-haemolytic transfusion reactions and decreasing the incidence of CMV disease. The use of recombinant growth factors remains controversial. There is no doubt that rh-GCSF and rh-GMCSF administered to patients post transplant reduces the length of neutropenia, especially in the autologous setting,[38] but their contribution to the overall outcome is difficult to estimate. Likewise, recombinant erythropoietin (EPO) has been shown to reduce the requirement for red cell concentrates.[39] There is no doubt, however, that myeloid growth factors are essential for the collection of haemopoietic stem cells for allogeneic PBSC SCT, and for mobilising PBSC prior to autografting. The introduction of rh-KGF (keratinocyte growth factor) may have a role in reducing the degree of mucosal bowel injury, subsequently decreasing morbidity in recipients of allogeneic or autologous SCT. Preliminary clinical trials have shown a decrease in the incidence of severe mucositis in patients undergoing autografting.[40] However, more extensive clinical trials are required to precisely define the role of this new growth factor in patients undergoing allo and auto SCT.

11.9.3 Infection

Bacterial infection in the post-transplant period is rarely life-threatening. The majority of SCT recipients are nursed in HEPA-filtered rooms until there is evidence of engraftment, although with reduced intensity conditioning some units are prepared to carry out this manoeuvre in a day–ward setting. The use of laminar airflow rooms is not essential for the majority of recipients of SCT. Viral and fungal infections remain a major problem, although the outcome for both continues to improve with the advent of antiviral and antifungal agents. A recent publication by EBMT shows that epidemics of infection may still occur in transplant units with deaths from fungal and viral infection still being significant.[41]

The clinical spectrum of herpes simplex infection, however, has been radically altered by the use of prophylactic and therapeutic Acyclovir. Prophylaxis and early diagnosis together with pre-emptive treatment have greatly improved the survival rates of patients with CMV infection, and CMV pneumonia is now much less common.[42] Two invasive fungal antigens (Galactomannan, PCR) are in widespread use, but neither have met with universal approval as a diagnostic test. High-dose CT remains a very useful investigation in the appropriate setting in neutropenic febrile patients. The choice of antifungal agents has significantly widened in recent years and includes liposomal amphotericin, azoles and newer drugs such as echinocandins. The problems of toxicity and a limited spectrum against emerging fungal pathogens remain. The high cost of many of these agents reduces their availability in many countries. Life-threatening fungal infections are commonly seen in the setting of refractory leukaemia and unresponsive GvHD, and are often the agonal event.

11.9.4 Graft–versus–host disease (GvHD)

Even in the context of HLA identical sibling SCT, a syndrome called graft–versus–host disease (GvHD) may occur. This syndrome occurs when immunologically competent cells in the graft recognise antigens in the recipient, causing a graft–versus–host reaction. For GvHD to occur in man, the following criteria are fulfilled:

1. The graft must contain immunocompetent cells.
2. The host must express antigens not found in the donor.
3. The host must not be able to mount an immune response.[43]

Experimental evidence suggests that acute GvHD develops in three phases: epithelial injury caused by the conditioning regimen, activation of donor lymphocytes by antigens presented by the recipient dendritic cells, and cell death induced by activated donor T cells, cytokines (such as TNF-α) and the cells of the immune system of the host. HLA disparity or differences in minor histocompatibility antigens between donor and recipient are the major predisposing factors. Other factors include the age of the donor and the recipient, sex-mismatched SCT (female donor into male recipient), the source of the transplanted haemopoietic stem cells, the intensity of the conditioning regimen, and prophylaxis against GvHD.[43]

In spite of better histocompatability matching and developments such as new drugs to prevent GvHD or the use of non-myeloablative stem cell transplants, GvHD continues to occur in more than half of the patients who undergo SCT, and is the main contributor to TRM. Traditionally, acute GvHD (aGvHD) occurs in the first hundred days following SCT, and chronic GvHD thereafter. With the advent of non-myeloablative stem cell transplant, it is clear that this division is artificial and is not helpful clinically. Many patients develop a syndrome identical to aGvHD after the hundredth day in the non-myeloablative transplant setting.

Cyclosporin, tacrolimus and methotrexate continue to be the main drugs used as prophylaxis against GvHD. Removal of T cells from the graft prior to SCT (T-cell depletion) results in a marked diminution in the rate of GvHD, but unfortunately is associated with a significant increase in rejection and leukaemia relapse, especially in patients receiving SCT for CML.[44] Different approaches to radiation, including low doses of total lymphoid radiation and anti-T-cell antibodies (antithymocyte globulin: ATG), have recently been evaluated both in the animal and human model and may have an impact on the incidences of GvHD following SCT.[45]

The mainstay of treatment of GvHD is corticosteroids, which may be associated with a 50% partial response rate and a 25% complete response. Although this treatment is considered standard in most SCT units, it has never been subjected to a randomised prospective trial. A number of monoclonal antibodies have been used in the treatment of established refractory GvHD but as yet none of them have been shown to be widely effective.

Chronic GvHD (cGvHD) usually occurs in the setting of pre-existing aGvHD but this is not so in all cases. When cGvHD is generalised it is invariably accompanied by immunosuppression, which is associated with infection and autoimmune phenomena including cytopenias that are difficult to treat.

11.9.5 Growth and fertility

Now that there are many long-term survivors of SCT, growth retardation and infertility have been identified as particularly distressing legacies of a 'successful outcome'. In pre-pubertal children growth is impaired and the effects of total body irradiation, specifically on spinal growth, often limit the response to growth hormones. Single fraction TBI is more inhibitive than fractionated irradiation. Delayed puberty is seen in boys and girls. TBI and busulphan result in ovarian failure. Symptoms of premature menopause may be alleviated by hormone replacement. In a small number of cases ovulatory function recovers following an interval of many years.[46] Oocyte preservation and *in vitro* fertilisation (IVF) have been successfully applied to small numbers of patients undergoing SCT. Although successful pregnancies have resulted, this form of therapy is not applicable to large numbers of patients and clearly is limited to females. Sperm cryopreservation prior to SCT again usually results in poor yields and successful pregnancies are uncommon. Patient-assessed outcome measurements of quality of life of long-term survivors frequently come close to those of the normal population.[47]

11.10 Future Directions

The number of patients receiving Allo and Auto SCT continues to increase worldwide. Improvements in HLA typing have undoubtedly helped us to select more appropriate donors; however, paradoxically it may reduce the donor pool. The use of UCBT will increase and efforts to expand numbers of stem cells *in vitro* will continue. The introduction of non-myeloablative SCT widened the spectrum of patients for whom SCT is being recommended. Its reduced toxicity will probably increase its usage for nonmalignant conditions. In older adults GvHD continues to remain a problem and even though GvHD rates may be lower than in the 'classical' SCT setting, many recipients have co-morbidity, thus limiting the long-term success of this approach.

The search for the pluripotent stem cell capable of establishing long-term adult haemopoiesis continues but research has indicated other therapeutic possibilities for haemopoietic stem cells such as in the repair of damaged myocardial tissue.

Support care and diagnosis of infectious complications continues to improve but infertility continues to be a major problem for the majority of SCT recipients. It is doubtful if current techniques of sperm or oocyte preservation will be ever widely available. Lastly and most importantly, SCT remains a complex and expensive manoeuvre and thus is denied to millions of individuals. Better efforts to improve access to health care internationally and increased understanding of the basic pathobiology of haematological disorders surely will help.

References

1. Jacobson, L.O. *et al.* (1949). Effect of Spleen Protection on Mortality Following X-Irradiation, *J Lab Clin Med*, **34**, 1538–1544.
2. Bortin, M.M. (1970). A Compendium of Reported Human Bone Marrow Transplants, *Transplantation*, **9**, 571–587.
3. Thomas, E.D. *et al.* (1975). Bone Marrow Transplantation, *New Engl J Med*, **292**, 832–843.
4. Orlic, D. and Bondin D.M. (1994). What Defines a Pluripotent Hematopoietic Stem Cell (PHSC): Will the Real PHSC Please Stand Up! *Blood*, **84**, 3991–3994.
5. Gianni, A.M. *et al.* (1989). Granulocyte-Macrophage Colony-Stimulating Factor to Harvest Circulating Haemopoietic Stem Cells for Autotransplantation, *Lancet*, **2**, 580–585.
6. Coutinho, L.H. *et al.* (1993). 'Clonal and Long-Term Cultures Using Human Bone Marrow' in Testa, N.G. and Molineux, G. (eds.), *Haemopoiesis: A Practical Approach*, Oxford University Press, New York pp. 75–105.

7. Sutherland, H.J. *et al.* (1990). Functional Characterization of Individual Human Hematopoietic Stem Cells Cultured at Limiting Dilution on Supportive Marrow Stromal Layers, *Proc Natl Acad Sci USA*, **87**, 3584–3588.

8. Krause, D.S. *et al.* (1996). CD34: Structure, Biology, and Clinical Utility, *Blood*, **87**, 1–13.

9. McCann, S.R. and Lawler, M. (1993). Mixed Chimaerism: Detection and Significance Following BMT, *Bone Marrow Transplant*, **11**, 91–95.

10. Kolb, H.J. and Bender-Götze, G. (1990). Late Complications after Allogeneic Bone Marrow Transplantation for Leukaemia, *Bone Marrow Transplant*, **6**, 61–72.

11. Kassim, A.A. *et al.* (2005). Reduced-Intensity Allogeneic Hematopoietic Stem Cell Transplantation for Acute Leukemias: 'What is the Best Recipe?' *Bone Marrow Transplant*, **36**, 565–574.

12. McCann, S.R. *et al.* (2005). Hemopoietic Chimerism Following Stem Cell Transplantation, *Transfus Apher Sci*, **32**, 55–61.

13. Kumar, L. and Goldman, J.M. (1993). Bone Marrow Transplantation for Patients Lacking an HLA Identical Sibling Donor, *Curr Opin Hematol*, pp. 234–239.

14. O'Riordan, J.R. *et al.* (1992). Probability of Finding a Compatible Sibling Donor for Bone Marrow Transplantation in Ireland, *Bone Marrow Transplant*, **9**, 27–30.

15. Beatty, P.G. *et al.* (1993). Marrow Transplantation from Unrelated Donors for Treatment of Hematologic Malignancies: Effect of Mismatching for One HLA Locus, *Blood*, **81**, 249–253.

16. Sierra, J. *et al.* (2000). Unrelated Donor Marrow Transplantation for Acute Myeloid Leukemia: An Update of the Seattle Experience, *Bone Marrow Transplant*, **26**, 397–404.

17. Deisseroth, A.B. *et al.* (1994). Genetic Marking Shows that Ph+ Cells Present in Autologous Transplants of Chronic Myelogenous Leukemia (CML) Contribute to Relapse after Autologous Bone Marrow in CML, *Blood*, **83**, 3068–3067.

18. JACIE, www.jacie.org.

19. Directive 2004/23/EC of the European Parliament and of the Council of 31 March 2004 on setting standards of quality and safety for the donation, procurement, testing, processing, preservation, storage and distribution of human tissues and cells.

20. Schmitz, N. *et al.* (1995). Primary Transplantation of Allogeneic Peripheral Blood Progenitor Cells Mobilized by Filgrastim (Granulocyte Colony-Stimulating Factor), *Blood*, **85(6)**, 1666–1672.

21. Gluckman, E. *et al.* (1989). Hematopoietic Reconstitution in a Patient with Fanconi's Anemia by Means of Umbilical-Cord Blood from an HLA-Identical Sibling, *New Engl J Med*, **321**, 1174–1178.

22. Gluckman, E. *et al.* (2005). Human Leukocyte Antigen Matching in Cord Blood Transplantation, *Semin Hematol*, **42**, 85–90.
23. Anderson, D. *et al.* (2003). A Comparison of Related Donor Peripheral Blood and Bone Marrow Transplants: Importance of Late-Onset Chronic Graft-Versus-Host Disease and Infections, *Biol Blood Marrow Transplant*, **9**, 52–59.
24. Remberger, M. *et al.* (2005). Increased Risk of Extensive Chronic Graft-Versus-Host Disease after Allogeneic Peripheral Blood Stem Cell Transplantation Using Unrelated Donors, *Blood*, **105**, 548–551.
25. Rochelle *et al.* (1997). Solid Cancers after Bone Marrow Transplantation, *New Engl J Med*, **336**, 897–904.
26. McCann, S. and Wright, E. (2003). Donor Leukaemia: Perhaps a More Common Occurrence than we Thought! *Bone Marrow Transplant*, **32**, 455–457.
27. Druker, B.J. *et al.* (2001). Activity of a Specific Inhibitor of the BCR-ABL Tyrosine Kinase in the Blast Crisis of Chronic Myeloid Leukemia and Acute Lymphoblastic Leukemia with the Philadelphia Chromosome, *New Engl J Med*, **344**, 1038–1042.
28. Zaucha, J.M. *et al.* (2005). Imatinib Therapy Prior to Myeloablative Allogeneic Stem Cell Transplantation, *Bone Marrow Transplant*, **36**, 417–424.
29. Bacigalupo, A. *et al.* (2000). Treatment of Acquired Severe Aplastic Anemia: Bone Marrow Transplantation Compared with Immunosuppressive Therapy: The European Group for Blood and Marrow Transplantation Experience, *Semin Hematol*, **37**, 69–80.
30. Zurlo, M.G. *et al.* (1989). Survival and Causes of Death in Thalassaemia Major, *Lancet*, **2**, 27–30.
31. Fischer, A. *et al.* (1990). European Experience of Bone-Marrow Transplantation for Severe Combined Immunodeficiency, *Lancet*, **336**, 850–854.
32. Gianni, A.M. *et al.* (1997). High-Dose Chemotherapy and Autologous Bone Marrow Transplantation Compared with MACOP-B In Aggressive B-Cell Lymphoma, *New Engl J Med*, **336**, 1290–1297.
33. Attal, M. *et al.* (1996). A Prospective, Randomized Trial of Autologous Bone Marrow Transplantation and Chemotherapy in Multiple Myeloma. Intergroupe Français du Myélome, *New Engl J Med*, **335**, 91–97.
34. Arnold, R. *et al.* (1986). Hemopoietic Reconstitution after Bone Marrow Transplantation, *Exp Haematol*, **14**, 271–277.
35. Anasetti, C. *et al.* (1989). Effect of HLA Compatibility on Engraftment of Bone Marrow Transplants in Patients with Leukemia or Lymphoma, *New Engl J Med*, **320**, 197–204.
36. Deeg, H.J. *et al.* (1998). Long-Term Outcome after Marrow Transplantation for Severe Aplastic Anemia, *Blood*, **91**, 3637–3645.
37. Champlin, R.E. *et al.* (1989). Graft Failure Following Bone Marrow Transplantation for Severe Aplastic Anemia: Risk Factors and Treatment Results, *Blood*, **73**, 606–613.

38. Sheridan, W.P. *et al.* (1989). Granulocyte Colony-Stimulating Factor and Neutrophil Recovery after High-Dose Chemotherapy and Autologous Bone Marrow Transplantation, *Lancet*, **2**, 891–895.

39. Link, H. *et al.* (1994). A Controlled Trial of Recombinant Human Erythropoietin after Bone Marrow Transplantation, *Blood*, **84**, 3227–3335.

40. Spielberger, R. *et al.* (2004). Palifermin for Oral Mucositis after Intensive Therapy for Hematologic Cancers, *New Engl J Med*, **351**, 2590–2598.

41. McCann, S. *et al.* (2004). Outbreaks of Infectious Diseases in Stem Cell Transplant Units: A Silent Cause of Death for Patients and Transplant Programmes, *Bone Marrow Transplant*, **33**, 519–529.

42. Emanuel, D. *et al.* (1988). Cytomegalovirus Pneumonia after Bone Marrow Transplantation Successfully Treated with the Combination of Ganciclovir and High-Dose Intravenous Immune Globulin, *Ann Int Med*, **109**, 777–782.

43. Socie, G. (2005). Graft-versus-Host Disease: From the Bench to the Bedside? *New Engl J Med*, **353**, 1396–1397.

44. Apperley, J.F. *et al.* (1986). Bone Marrow Transplantation for Patients with Chronic Mycloid Leukaemia: T-Cell Depletion with Campath-1 Reduces the Incidence of Graft versus-Host Disease but May Increase the Risk of Leukaemic Relapse, *Bone Marrow Transplant*, **1**, 53–66.

45. Lowsky, R. *et al.* (2005). Protective Conditioning for Acute Graft-versus-Host Disease, *N Engl J Med*, **353**, 1321–1331.

46. Sanders, J.E. *et al.* (1991). The Impact of Marrow Transplant Preparative Regimens on Subsequent Growth and Development. The Seattle Marrow Transplant Team, *Semin Haematol*, **28**, 244–249.

47. Hayden, P.J. *et al.* (2004). A Single-Centre Assessment of Long-Term Quality-of-Life Status after Sibling Allogeneic Stem Cell Transplantation for Chronic Myeloid Leukaemia in First Chronic Phase, *Bone Marrow Transplant*, **34**, 545–556.

Recent Advances in Immunosuppressive Drugs in Organ Transplantation

Anthony N. Warrens

12.1 Introduction

The world used to be a much simpler place! When organ replacement was first established as a routine medical procedure (with renal transplantation in the 1960s), the unquestioned standard immunosuppressive regime (indeed, the only effective immunosuppressive regime) was a combination of corticosteroids and azathioprine (Imuran). It was only in the years around 1980 that there was a significant advance with the introduction of the new calcineurin inhibitor (CNI), ciclosporin (spelled differently then!) and two types of antibody preparation: polyclonal anti-lymphocyte preparations (anti-lymphocyte globulin and anti-thymocyte globulin) and the monoclonal anti-CD3ε T cell agent, OKT3 (now officially called muronomab). All three, but ciclosporin in particular, made a significant contribution to immunosuppression. By the early 1990s, the internationally accepted standard immunosuppressive regime consisted of corticosteroids, azathioprine and ciclosporin. There was some variation in the use of the new antibody preparations: in the United States there was a tendency to use them more routinely; in Europe, they tended to be reserved for highly immunological risk situations.

There was a modest improvement in ciclosporin's pharmacokinetics after the macroemulsion Sandimmune was replaced by the microemulsion Neoral. But apart from this, for the next decade and a half, efforts were focused on how best to use these agents: for example, what did you do with ciclosporin when there was a high risk of ischaemia or actual delayed graft function? When should you use an antibody preparation, and which one? What were the appropriate ciclosporin levels to aim for?

However, between 1995 and 2000, there was an explosion of new agents that became available as new immunosuppressive drugs:

1. Tacrolimus, an alternative CNI to ciclosporin that was sufficiently different, chemically, to raise hopes that it was not just a 'me-too' alternative.
2. A range of new anti-metabolites to rival azathioprine, of which the first was the mycophenolic acid (MPA) pro-drug, mycophenolate mofetil (MMF; Cellcept). More recently, an alternative MPA pro-drug has been developed: mycophenolate sodium (MPS; Certican). While these agents (and almost exclusively MMF) have captured the 'alternative anti-metabolite' market in Europe and North America, other anti-metabolites such as brequinar and leflunamide-derivatives have been used in other parts of the world.
3. A large number of antibody preparations targeting various populations and sub-populations of leucocytes, building on the evident success of the polyclonal anti-lymphocyte preparations and OKT3. In recent years, many of these have aimed to diminish the adverse effects of infusing non-human protein, by taking advantage of new recombinant DNA technology. As a result, these antibodies have been chimaeric (in which the constant immunoglobulin domains have been replaced with human-constant immunoglobulin domains, leaving only the variable domains containing the antigen-binding sites as the only non-human constituents of the protein) or even humanised (in which only the three hypervariable [complementarity-determining] regions of the mouse variable domains — the protein loops that actually contact the antigen — are of non-human origin). Only three have come into clinical practice: basiliximab (Simulect), daclizumab (Zenepax) and alemtuzumab (Campath-1H).
4. A group of drugs with a new mechanism of action, the inhibition of mTOR (mammalian target of rapamycin), of which (unsurprisingly

given the name of its target) rapamycin is the clinical prototype. More recently, its name has changed to sirolimus (SRL). A closely related drug, originally referred to as rapamycin–derivative (RAD), but now known as everolimus (Certican), has also been developed.

12.2 Mechanisms of Action of Currently Used Immunosuppressive Agents

While all the drugs currently used in the clinical practice of immunosuppression in transplantation have a number of mechanisms of action (some desirable, others not), they all share the fact that they have some impact on the activation process of the CD4+ T lymphocyte. The CD4+ T cell is central to the initiation of an immune response. Without the 'help' provided by this cell (also known as the 'helper T cell') in recruiting the different effector arms of the immune response, there would be a severely curtailed immunological response to transplanted tissue. Indeed, the current agents attack the activation process at a series of different levels. Since no drug is 100% effective, the use of agents with sequential inhibitory action is an efficient approach. In addition, it allows for the minimisation of exposure to each agent, thus reducing the agent-specific (as opposed to the immunosuppression-specific) adverse effects.

12.3 The Deployment of New Immunosuppressive Agents in Clinical Practice

As outlined above, there has been a veritable explosion in new therapeutic options in this therapeutic area over the short period of approximately a decade. Hence it has not been possible to study each new development sequentially. As a result, a number of competing strategies for immunosuppression have developed. The rest of this chapter will examine the place of each new class of drugs in the therapeutic armamentarium, looking at how they have been deployed in each of the competing strategies. In order to avoid complexity, the chapter will largely focus on the use of these drugs in renal transplantation.

12.4 Tacrolimus (Prograf)

Tacrolimus found a place in liver transplantation much earlier than it did in kidney transplantation. In part, this was due to the hope that, as an alternative CNI, it would show lower levels of nephrotoxicity than ciclosporin. In fact, there is no difference between the two agents with respect to nephrotoxicity. Indeed, for a time it proved difficult to demonstrate any differences in efficacy between the two. It was clear that they differed in their adverse-effect profiles (except with respect to nephrotoxicity): ciclosporin had more marked skin and gum side effects, particularly hirsuitism and gingival hyperplasia; by contrast, tacrolimus had a greater tendency to cause impaired glucose tolerance. More recently, it also became clear that ciclosporin induced a greater increase in hyperlipidaemia and hypertension than tacrolimus. Initial studies comparing the immunosuppressive efficacy of the two agents were difficult to interpret because they compared tacrolimus with the macroemulsion preparation of ciclosporin, Sandimmune. Since that preparation is no longer generally supplied, these studies are principally of historical interest.

More recently, a number of studies comparing tacrolimus with the microemulsion preparation of ciclosporin (Neoral) have been undertaken. These were summarised in a meta-analysis that demonstrated clear superiority of tacrolimus over ciclosporin in terms of graft survival (relative risk for tacrolimus at three years: 0.71 [95% confidence intervals 0.52–0.96; $p < 0.03$]) and steroid-resistant acute rejection (relative risk for tacrolimus at one year: 0.49 [95% confidence intervals 0.37–0.64; $p < 0.00001$]).[1] This study also highlighted the differences in adverse effects between the two agents, for example, the increased risk in new requirement for insulin on tacrolimus relative to ciclosporin (3.84 [95% confidence intervals 2.01–7.41; $p < 0.0001$]).

In the light of this data, it is unsurprising that tacrolimus has now become the dominant CNI. There does remain a role for cyclosporine, not only for stable patients already receiving the drug but also for patients who do not need the increased potency of tacrolimus, and for those in whom it is advisable to minimise the risks of the tacrolimus-specific adverse effects.

As the effectiveness of therapeutic regimens has increased, the focus has moved from the prevention of acute rejection to the avoidance of what are now the two commonest causes of the loss of the kidney transplant: death of the recipient with a functioning graft and chronic allograft damage. The dominant causes of death of the recipients are cardiovascular, and CNIs increase the risk of cardiovascular disease by exacerbating hypertension and hyperlipidaemia. Similarly, CNIs contribute directly through their nephro-toxic effects to the chronic damage that has often been described as chronic allograft nephropathy (CAN), although that term is now no longer used.

Accordingly, the focus of therapeutic development at the moment is on minimising the exposure of patients to long-term CNIs. The availability of a new range of more potent alternative immunosuppressive agents has made that possible. This will be discussed further below.

12.5 Anti-Metabolites

The only new agent in this class to have made a significant impact in the clinical practice of transplantation is mycophenolate mofetil (MMF). Like azathioprine, MMF is an inhibitor of purine synthesis; but unlike azathio-prine, it is a non-competitive inhibitor of one of the enzymes of the purine synthetic pathway (inosine monophosphate dehydrogenase: IMPDH). The early studies of ciclosporin-treated patients demonstrate that it had greater efficacy than either placebo or azathioprine, as judged by prevalence of acute rejection of graft failure in the first year following transplantation in three trials of 1,493 patients.[2] The six-month treatment failure rate was lower on MMF than placebo (30% versus 56%) in the European study,[3] and lower on MMF than azathiprone in the Tricontinental Study (38% versus 50%)[4] and the US Study (31% versus 48%).[5] Three-year analysis showed ongoing ben-efit in the comparison of MMF with placebo,[6] but not with azathioprine,[7,8] although the studies were not aimed at detecting benefits that long after transplantation.

As mentioned above, there is currently a major move to decrease patients' exposure to CNIs. It has been shown that the increased potency of MMF over azathioprine allows the use of lower doses of CNI. A recent study of 1,645 patients has shown that usage of MMF (plus daclizumab) allows lower exposure to either cicloporin or tacrolimus, and produces better out-comes in terms of graft function and rejection when compared with more conventional doses of ciclosporin or even sirolimus.[9] It remains unclear how this approach will be taken up.

12.6 Newer Monoclonal Antibodies

Both basiliximab and daclizumab have proven to be very effective induction agents. The initial studies on each showed a significant effect on acute rejection. Basiliximab showed a reduction in acute rejection at 6 months from 44% to 30%,[10] and daclizumab showed a reduction in acute rejection, over the same period, from 47% to 28%.[11] They are particularly attractive agents since they have been shown to have an extremely safe adverse-effects profile. Also, they are very inexpensive compared to other immunosuppressive agents as they are only administered at the beginning of the life of the transplant, not as long-term ongoing agents. For this reason, basiliximab and daclizumab found particular favour in the cost-effectiveness analysis of immunosuppressive drugs in renal transplantation undertaken by the UK's National Institute for Health and Clinical Excellence (NICE).

The role of alemtuzumab (Campath-1H) is not yet as well established. A number of studies have confirmed its efficacy, although there is, as yet, no unanimity on the immunosuppressive context in which it should be administered. Its use with sirolimus alone was associated with an unacceptably high incidence of acute rejection,[12] but the use of alemtuzumab with a CNI, MMF and steroids, when compared with an anti-CD25 antibody, anti-thymocyte globulin or other antibody treatment, resulted in less rejection and (in those with delayed graft function) improved graft survival.[13] There were some concerns with the level of adverse effects associated with over-immunosuppression and an anxiety that the prolonged depletion of white cells following the use of alemtuzumab may merely delay the onset of rejection. In the Imperial College Healthcare NHS Trust, where alemtuzumab plus low-dose tacrolimus is being compared with daclizumab, as well as standard tacrolimus plus MMF (n = 217 to date), both groups had been found to have very good graft survival (98.4% and 95.3%, respectively, at 24 months) and a low prevalence of rejection (rejection-free survival of 86.2% and 86.0% at 24 months). None of the problems outlined above have been noticed.[14]

12.7 Sirolimus (Rapamycin)

mTOR is responsible for activating the cell cycle, and thus cellular proliferation. Without this proliferation, even if it recognises alloantigen, a CD4+ T lymphocyte will not be activated. mTOR is inhibited by sirolimus.

The role of sirolimus in the therapeutic approach to renal transplantation remains unclear. Initial studies considered a role for sirolimus as a potential alternative adjunct to therapy to either azathioprine or MMF. It is clear that, in the context of ciclosporin and steroids, it offers superior immunosuppression over placebo. A study of 576 patients showed a six-month acute rejection rate of 25% in patients receiving sirolimus 2 mg/kg, compared to 42% in the placebo arm (p < 0.001), and a rate of steroid-resistant rejection of 4% and 8%, respectively (p = 0.004).[14] Another study, involving 719 patients, showed that the same dose of sirolimus was superior to azathioprine, also in patients receiving ciclosporin and steroids: the acute rejection rate was 17% and 30%, respectively (p = 0.002).[15,16] But a much larger registry report, involving 23,016 patients, suggested that sirolimus is less potent than MMF, with a one-year acute rejection rate (in 2000) of 21% of patients on sirolimus and 16% of those on MMF (p = 0.007).[17] Indeed, that same report showed that the MMF arm had superior four-year graft survival (79%) than the sirolimus arm (75%) (p = 0.002). Similar data have been observed in a comparison of sirolimus with MMF in patients receiving tacrolimus and steroids (n = 361): the one-year creatinine was 1.5 mg/dL in the sirolimus arm and 1.3 mg/dL in the MMF arm (p = 0.03).[18]

However, there has been more interest in using sirolimus to minimise exposure to CNIs. In a European study of 83 patients receiving azathioprine and steroids, sirolimus was compared directly with ciclosporin and found to have a comparable 12-month graft survival and rates of acute rejection, but lower three-month creatinine levels (127 mcmol/L compared with 167 mcmol/L), although the difference in creatinine levels was no longer significant at 12 months.[19] In a North American study of 61 patients receiving MMF and steroids plus induction basiliximab, sirolimus was compared with ciclosporin and showed similar rejection rates, but a difference in creatinine that was maintained at 12 months (1.93 mg/dL compared with 1.32 mg/dL), a significant difference in glomerular filtration rate at two years (49 mL/min versus 61 mL/min), and a much higher percentage of patients with Banff grade 0 on biopsy at two years (67% versus 21%).[20,21] A similar study in which 165 patients received MMF and steroids compared sirolimus with tacrolimus and showed no difference in rejection rates or glomerular filtration rate, but did note a lower prevalence of chronic vascular changes on biopsy in the sirolimus group (26% compared with 43%).[22]

However, there are significant adverse events associated with sirolimus use, particularly in the early post-operative phase, such as poor wound healing and prolonged lymphocoeles. In addition, the concern about CNI exposure is with the chronic effects rather than short-term exposure. Accordingly, other studies have focused on the use of sirolimus to permit the staged reduction or withdrawal of CNI dose under sirolimus cover, often introduced with a raised dose in a staged fashion. A systematic review of six trials, involving 1,047 patients, reported that CNI-withdrawal from a sirolimus-based regime was associated with an increased risk of acute rejection (6% risk difference p = 0.002) but a higher creatinine clearance (difference 7.5 mL/mon; p < 0.00001) and no difference in graft loss or death at one year.[23]

12.8 Corticosteroids

In the light of the well-recognised long-term complications of steroid therapy and the need to minimise the use of agents that exacerbate risk factors for cardiovascular disease, over recent years there has been a major drive to minimise, withdraw or even eliminate the use of steroids in transplant recipients. Early attempts to do so had been associated with an unacceptably high risk of graft rejection and, in fact, a large meta-analysis of the effect of steroid withdrawal on 1,984 patients did show a significant deleterious effect (relative risk 1.38 [95% confidence intervals 1.08–1.67]).[24] A more recent report involving 1,681 patients, albeit including data dating back to 1984, showed something similar.[25] However, more recently, a large number of studies have been published that have demonstrated that it is possible to withdraw steroids under cover of the newer, more potent immunosuppressive regimens described in Sections 12.4 to 12.7.[26−29]

12.9 Conclusions

The range of therapeutic options now available for immunosuppression in the transplant recipient is much broader than it has ever been. It is no longer possible to talk about a 'standard' regime, as was the case only ten years ago. In part, this is because of the increasing realisation that the needs of individual patients vary. Firstly, it is possible to begin to quantify the level of immunogenic challenge a particular graft represents: is it well matched? Has there been a long cold-ischaemic time? Is the recipient sensitised? In addition, the appropriateness of a given regime for a particular individual can be judged: would one wish to give someone at risk of diabetes the more diabetogenic CNI, tacrolimus? Is the proposed total burden of immunosuppression too great given the patient's historical exposure to these drugs and their current clinical state?

But in addition to differing patient demands, there are increasing options for varying immunosuppression agents. Some trends are very clear: there is a high level of enthusiasm for minimising and eliminating steroids from the regime as soon as is feasible. In addition, there is a strong desire to minimise CNI exposure with a view to decreasing chronic nephrotoxicity. However, there are several immunosuppressive contexts in which this may be done. Which of those outlined above will achieve pole position remains to be seen. It is an interesting time in the field of immunosuppression.

References

1. Webster, A.C. *et al.* (2005). Tacrolimus versus Ciclosporin as Primary Immunosuppression for Kidney Transplant Recipients: Meta-Analysis and Meta-Regression of Randomised Trial Data, *BMJ*, **331(7520)**, 810.
2. Halloran, P. *et al.* (1997). The International Mycophenolate Mofetil Renal Transplant Study Groups. Mycophenolate Mofetil in Renal Allograft Recipients: A Pooled Efficacy Analysis of Three Randomized, Double-Blind, Clinical Studies in Prevention of Rejection, *Transplantation*, **63(1)**, 39–47.
3. European Mycophenolate Mofetil Cooperative Study Group (1995). Placebo-Controlled Study of Mycophenolate Mofetil Combined with Cyclosporin and Corticosteroids for Prevention of Acute Rejection, *Lancet*, **345(8961)**, 1321–1325.
4. The Tricontinental Mycophenolate Mofetil Renal Transplantation Study Group. (1996). A Blinded, Randomized Clinical Trial of Mycophenolate Mofetil for the Prevention of Acute Rejection in Cadaveric Renal Transplantation, *Transplantation*, **61(7)**, 1029–1037.
5. Sollinger, H.W. *et al.* (U.S. Renal Transplant Mycophenolate Mofetil Study Group). (1995). Mycophenolate Mofetil for the Prevention of Acute Rejection

in Primary Cadaveric Renal Allograft Recipients, *Transplantation*, **60(3)**, 225–232.

6. European Mycophenolate Mofetil Cooperative Study Group. (1999). Mycophenolate Mofetil in Renal Transplantation: 3-Year Results from the Placebo-Controlled Trial, *Transplantation*, **68(3)**, 391–396.

7. Mathew, T.H. (Tricontinental Mycophenolate Mofetil Renal Transplantation Study Group). (1998). A Blinded, Long-Term, Randomized Multicenter Study of Mycophenolate Mofetil in Cadaveric Renal Transplantation: Results at Three Years, *Transplantation*, **65(11)**, 1450–1454.

8. US Renal Transplant Mycophenolate Mofetil Study Group. (1999). Mycophenolate Mofetil in Cadaveric Renal Transplantation, *Am J Kidney Dis*, **34(2)**, 296–303.

9. Ekberg, H. *et al.* (2006). Symphony — Comparing Standard Immunosuppression to Low-Dose Cyclosporine, Tacrolimus or Sirolimus in Combination with MMF, Daclizumab and Corticosteroids in Renal Transplantation, *Am J Transplant*, **6(S2)**, 83 (Abstract).

10. Nashan, B. *et al.* (1997). Randomised Trial of Basiliximab Versus Placebo for Control of Acute Cellular Rejection in Renal Allograft Recipients, CHIB 201 International Study Group. *Lancet*, **350(9086)**, 1193–1198.

11. Vincenti, F. *et al.* (1998). Interleukin-2-receptor Blockade with Daclizumab to Prevent Acute Rejection in Renal Transplantation, Daclizumab Triple Therapy Study Group, *New Engl J Med*, **338(3)**, 161–165.

12. Barth, R.N. *et al.* (2006). Outcomes at 3 Years of a Prospective Pilot Study of Campath-1H and Sirolimus Immunosuppression for Renal Transplantation, *Transpl Int*, **19(11)**, 885–892.

13. Knechtle, S.J. *et al.* (2004). Campath-1H in Renal Transplantation: The University of Wisconsin Experience, *Surgery*, **136(4)**, 754–670.

14. Chan, E. (2008). Personal communication.

15. MacDonald, A.S. (2001). A Worldwide, Phase III, Randomized, Controlled, Safety and Efficacy Study of a Sirolimus/Cyclosporine Regimen for Prevention of Acute Rejection in Recipients of Primary Mismatched Renal Allografts, *Transplantation*, **71(2)**, 271–280.

16. Kahan, B.D. (2000). Efficacy of Sirolimus Compared with Azathioprine for Reduction of Acute Renal Allograft Rejection: A Randomised Multicentre Study, The Rapamune US Study Group, *Lancet*, **356(9225)**, 194–202.

17. Meier-Kriesche, H.U. *et al.* (2004). Sirolimus with Neoral versus Mycophenolate Mofetil with Neoral is Associated with Decreased Renal Allograft Survival, *Am J Transplant*, **4(12)**, 2058–2066.

18. Mendez, R. *et al.* (2005). A Prospective, Randomized Trial of Tacrolimus in Combination with Sirolimus or Mycophenolate Mofetil in Kidney Transplantation: Results at 1 Year, *Transplantation*, **80(3)**, 303–309.

19. Groth, C.G. *et al.* (1999). Sirolimus (Rapamycin)-Based Therapy in Human Renal Transplantation: Similar Efficacy and Different Toxicity Compared with

Cyclosporine, Sirolimus European Renal Transplant Study Group, *Transplantation*, **67(7)**, 1036–1042.

20. Flechner, S.M. *et al.* (2002). Kidney Transplantation without Calcineurin Inhibitor Drugs: A Prospective, Randomized Trial of Sirolimus Versus Cyclosporine, *Transplantation*, **74(8)**, 1070–1076.
21. Flechner, S.M. *et al.* (2004). De Novo Kidney Transplantation Without Use of Calcineurin Inhibitors Preserves Renal Structure and Function at Two Years, *Am J Transplant*, **4(11)**, 1776–1785.
22. Larson, T.S. *et al.* (2006). Complete Avoidance of Calcineurin Inhibitors in Renal Transplantation: A Randomized Trial Comparing Sirolimus and Tacrolimus, *Am J Transplant*, **6(3)**, 514–522.
23. Mulay, A.V. *et al.* (2005). Calcineurin Inhibitor Withdrawal From Sirolimus-Based Therapy in Kidney Transplantation: A Systematic Review of Randomized Trials, *Am J Transplant*, **5(7)**, 1748–1756.
24. Kasiske, B.L. *et al.* (2000). A Meta-Analysis of Immunosuppression Withdrawal Trials in Renal Transplantation, *J Am Soc Nephrol*, **11(10)**, 1910–1917.
25. Tan, J.Y. *et al.* (2006). Steroid Withdrawal Increases Risk of Acute Rejection But Reduces Infection: A Meta-Analysis of 1681 Cases in Renal Transplantation, *Transplant Proc*, **38(7)**, 2054–2056.
26. Kumar, M.S. *et al.* (2006). Safety and Efficacy of Steroid Withdrawal Two Days After Kidney Transplantation: Analysis of Results at Three Years, *Transplantation*, **81(6)**, 832–839.
27. Wlodarczyk, Z. *et al.* (2005). Steroid Withdrawal at 3 Months after Kidney Transplantation: A Comparison of Two Tacrolimus-Based Regimens, *Transpl Int*, **18(2)**, 157–162.
28. ter Meulen, C.G. *et al.* (2004). Steroid Withdrawal at 3 Days after Renal Transplantation with Anti-IL-2 Receptor Alpha Therapy: A Prospective, Randomized, Multicenter Study, *Am J Transplant*, **4(5)**, 803–810.
29. Boots, J.M. *et al.* (2002). Early Steroid Withdrawal in Renal Transplantation with Tacrolimus Dual Therapy: A Pilot Study, *Transplantation*, **74(12)**, 1703–1709.

Index

237